WH 140 DAV

# Starting to Read ECGs

## DATE DUE

| 16/ 9/19 | |
|---|---|
| | |
| | |
| | |
| | |
| | |
| | |
| | |
| | |
| | |
| | |
| | |
| | |
| | |
| | |
| | |
| | PRINTED IN U.S.A. |

Alan Davies • Alwyn Scott

# Starting to Read ECGs

A Comprehensive Guide
to Theory and Practice

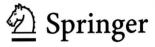 Springer

Alan Davies
School of Computer Science
University of Manchester
Manchester
UK

Alwyn Scott
Cardiology High Dependency Unit
Papworth Hospital NHS Foundation Trust
Cambridge
UK

ISBN 978-1-4471-4964-4       ISBN 978-1-4471-4965-1   (eBook)
DOI 10.1007/978-1-4471-4965-1
Springer London Heidelberg New York Dordrecht

Library of Congress Control Number: 2014956281

Springer is part of Springer Science+Business Media (www.springer.com)

*This book is dedicated to the memory of:*
Bruce Nigel Davies
1953–2013

# Preface

This book is the second in a series of books aimed at introducing the electrocardiogram (ECG) to practitioners whose roles incorporate some level of ECG interpretation. This book expands on some of the topics introduced in the first book of the series but offers a deeper perspective, with more detailed background information and a variety of practical interpretation methods that the user is free to choose from and apply to their clinical practice.

The authors have also endeavored to introduce several new topics including an introduction to the pediatric ECG and genetic cardiac conditions in an attempt to deepen readers' awareness of some of the broader clinical issues.

This book can be read as a standalone book by those who already possess some basic ECG knowledge and wish to deepen and expand their knowledge base or by those who have read the first book in the series and wish to consolidate and expand on what they have already read.

The book uses lots of diagrams, tables summarizing key points, and practical examples to reinforce learning and summarize information succinctly. We hope you will find this book a useful addition in your continuing journey to master the ECG.

Manchester, UK                                                              Alan Davies

# Authors

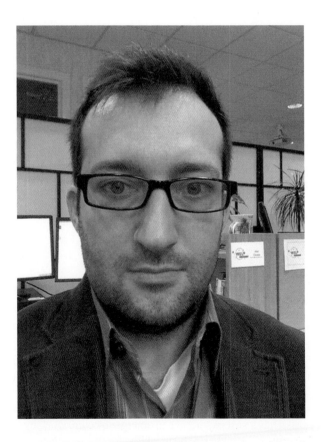

**Alan Davies** graduated from Birmingham City University with a first class honours degree and a postgraduate degree module in ECGs and arrhythmias. Alan was also awarded a first place prize for adult nursing students in the inaugural Health Care Awards. Alan went on to work in cardiac catheterisation, gaining experience in routine and emergency angiograms including primary PCI. Alan has also assisted in pacemaker/AICD insertion, transoesopheageal echo (TOE), cardioversion and electrophysiological studies. Alan is currently a PhD student combining his knowledge and interests in computer science and electrocardiograms by carrying out research into capturing expertise through the observation of visual behaviour and using eye-tracking technology to improve aspects of human and computer ECG interpretation.

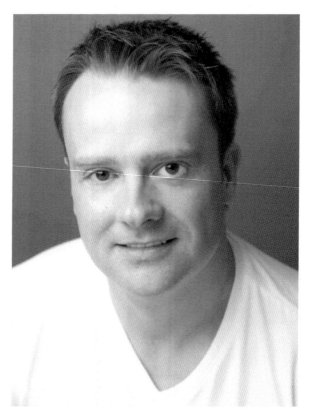

**Alwyn Scott** graduated from Birmingham University and has worked in the NHS since 1995. He is currently employed as senior staff nurse for the Cardiology High Dependency Department at Papworth Hospital in Cambridgeshire. His role is predominantly that of working with patients who are in acute stages of having heart attacks both pre- and post-primary PCI. Alwyn is also heavily involved in staff education. Alongside specialist knowledge in acute cardiac nursing and ECG interpretation, Alwyn also has a vast experience in emergency care, working in accident and emergency departments and also in the front line for the ambulance service responding to 999 calls.

# Acknowledgments

We would like to thank the following for their help, support, and encouragement in the writing of this book:

Vicki Jephcote

Monika Golaś

Victoria John PhD

# Contents

# Chapter 1
# Cardiac Anatomy and Electrophysiology

**Keywords** Anatomy • Physiology • Electrophysiology • Action potential • Depolarization • Repolarization • Cardiac output • Blood pressure • Circulatory system

## Background

The human heart is an organ that has both mechanical and electrical components. Both knowledge of basic cardiac anatomy and physiology, as well as electrophysiology is necessary to fully understand the basics of the electrocardiogram (ECG). Understanding and awareness of these elements in the normal heart is essential before building a more complete picture of the pathological heart.

We will start with an overview of the basic anatomy and physiology of the heart before looking more specifically at the electrophysiological components of the heart's function. Finally we will look at how the mechanical and electrical systems of the heart interact with each other in a healthy individual.

## Anatomy of the Heart

Figure 1.1 displays the main anatomical features of the human heart. A brief description of some of the primary anatomical features follows.

### *Chambers*

The heart consists of four chambers, two small chambers located superiorly, called the left and right atrium and two larger chambers located inferiorly called the left and right ventricle. The left ventricle is larger than the right as it has to pump blood to the majority of the body, whereas the right ventricle pumps blood into the lungs. The atria and ventricles are separated from one another by the interatrial septum and the interventricular septum respectively.

© Springer-Verlag London 2015
A. Davies, A. Scott, *Starting to Read ECGs: A Comprehensive Guide
to Theory and Practice*, DOI 10.1007/978-1-4471-4965-1_1

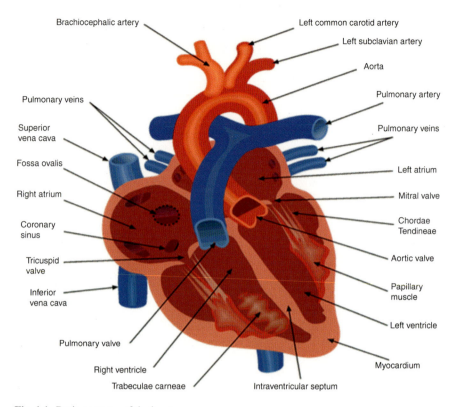

**Fig. 1.1**  Basic anatomy of the heart

## *Valves*

The heart also has four valves. The tricuspid and mitral valves, known as the atrio-ventricular valves as they sit between the atria and ventricles allowing access for blood to pass from the atria to the ventricles. The other two valves are the aortic and pulmonary valves, and are referred to as the semilunar valves which lead to the aorta and the pulmonary artery. The principle purpose of the valves is to prevent regurgitation of blood from the ventricles back into the atria. The valves open when the pressure in the chamber filled with blood exceeds the pressure in the area past the valve. For example when the pressure in the right atrium exceeds the pressure in the right ventricle, the valve opens and the blood passes from atrium to ventricle.

The valves have flaps that are sometimes referred to as leaflets or cusps. The tricuspid valve has three such flaps or cusps. The mitral valve is also referred to as the bicuspid valve and has two cusps.

## Chordae Tendineae

The chordae tendineae are fibrous tendon like cords that connect to the tricuspid valve in the right ventricle and the mitral valve in the left ventricle. When the valves close the chordae tendineae prevent the cusps from swinging upwards into the atrial cavity.

## Fossa Ovalis

The fossa ovalis is the remains of what was once a hole (foramen) that existed between the left atrium and the right atrium, located in the atrial septum. This hole allows blood to bypass the lungs in a developing fetus when fetal oxygen supply is provided via the placenta, as the fetal lungs are undeveloped.

## Trabeculae Carneae

The trabeculae carneae are muscular columns of irregular shape that exist in both ventricles. In the left ventricle they are smooth and fine when compared to those in the right ventricle. It is believed that the function of the trabeculae carneae is to prevent suction that could impair the pumping action of the ventricles that could otherwise occur if the ventricles were smooth. When the trabeculae carneae contract they inturn pull on the chordae tendineae.

## Papillary Muscle

A type of trabeculae carneae that are connected to ventricular surface at one end and at the other to the chordae tendineae.

## Coronary Sinus

The coronary sinus allows the cardiac veins carrying deoxygenated blood to drain into the right atrium.

## The Great Vessels

Incorporate the vena cava, pulmonary artery/veins and the aorta. In the rest of the body oxygenated blood is found in arteries and deoxygenated blood in the veins. This general rule does not apply to the heart, which sometimes causes confusion. The pulmonary artery carries deoxygenated blood into the lungs and the pulmonary veins carry the resulting oxygenated blood into the left atrium. The aorta trifurcates into three other branches; brachiocephalic, left common carotid and left subclavian arteries which supply the upper portion of the body with blood. The descending aorta bifurcates into the common iliac arteries supplying the legs with blood.

## Heart Wall

The wall of the heart (Fig. 1.2) is made up of several layers. The innermost layer is the endocardium, followed by the thicker myocardium that makes up the cardiac muscle and consists of cardiomyocytes, which are cardiac muscle cells. The outer layer of the heart wall is known as the epicardium. Directly following the epicardium is a gap called the pericardial cavity that separates the heart from the pericardium. The pericardial cavity contains pericardial (serous) fluid. The pericardium is a protective membrane that covers the heart and also envelops the roots of the great cardiac vessels. The principle functions of the pericardium (Fig. 1.3) are to anchor the heart in place preventing excess movement, act as a barrier to protect the heart from internal infection from other organs and to lubricate the heart.

## Circulatory Function of the Heart

Deoxygenated blood is emptied into the right atrium via the vena cava. The inferior vena cava returns blood from the lower portion of the body as the superior vena cava

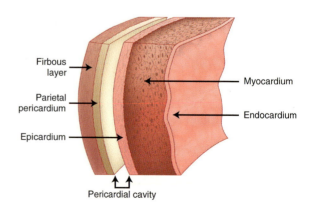

**Fig. 1.2** Layers of the heart from outside to inside

**Fig. 1.3** The pericardium

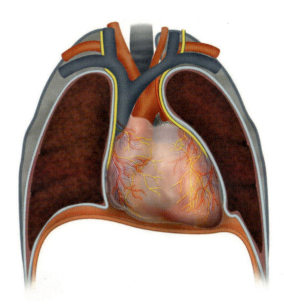

returns blood from the higher portion. Blood is then pumped through the tricuspid valve into the right ventricle and into the lungs via the pulmonary artery where it is oxygenated. Oxygenated blood then returns from the lungs into the left atrium where it can be pumped to the rest of the body by the left ventricle, via the aorta. The circulatory system has two divisions; the systemic and pulmonary circulatory system (Fig. 1.4). The pulmonary system is responsible for circulating blood from the right ventricle to the lungs and back into the left atrium. The systemic system as the name implies pumps blood via the aorta to every other part of the body. This is why the left ventricle is larger and more powerful than the right, as it has to pump blood over greater distances. This is also why left ventricular pressure is higher than right ventricular pressure.

## *Coronary Arteries*

In addition to the heart pumping blood to the rest of the body, the heart itself requires its own blood supply in order to function as an organ. As blood is pumped via the aorta to the rest of the body, it also passes into the coronary arteries that are located at the aortic root. There are two main coronary arteries, called the left and right coronary arteries respectively (Fig. 1.5). The left coronary artery bifurcates into the circumflex and left anterior descending arteries. Deoxygenated blood is returned to the right ventricle by coronary veins via the coronary sinus. The coronary arteries are discussed in more detail in Chap. 7.

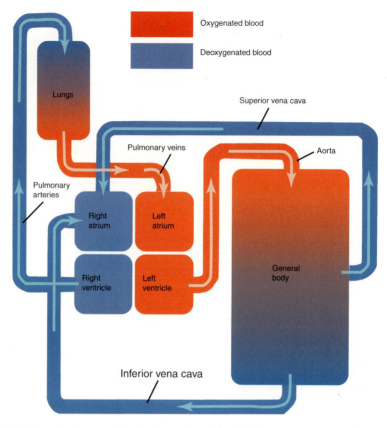

**Fig. 1.4** Schematic diagram of the circulatory function of the heart

## Starling's Law of the Heart

The Frank Starling law essentially states that an increase in end diastolic volume corresponds with an increase in the hearts stroke volume. To put it another way the greater the degree of stretch to the cardiac muscle in diastole (relaxation of cardiac muscle), the greater the force of contraction in systole (contraction of cardiac muscle). What goes in comes out. Problems can occur if the heart is continually maximally stretched for a long period of time, as occurs in heart failure. Like an elastic band, if it is continually maximally stretched it will become weak, lose elasticity and fail to return to it's original shape.

## Preload and Afterload

The heart's preload and afterload are important factors in determining the stroke volume. Preload refers to the amount of muscular tension when the ventricle contracts at the end of diastole to eject the blood from the filled ventricle. Afterload is therefore the systemic vascular resistance the left ventricle pushes against in order to expel the blood during systole (Fig. 1.6).

**Fig. 1.5** Coronary arteries

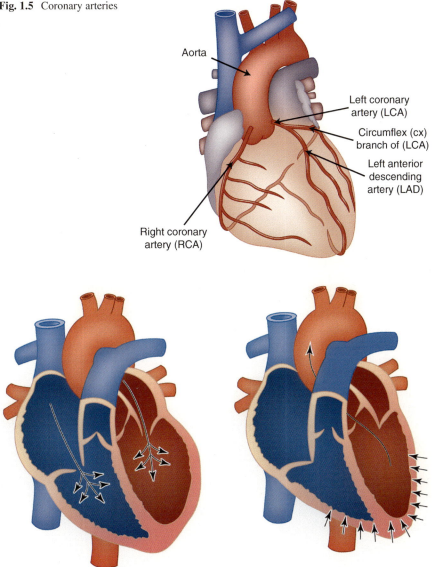

Aorta

Left coronary
artery (LCA)

Circumflex (cx)
branch of (LCA)

Left anterior
descending
artery (LAD)

Right coronary
artery (RCA)

**Fig. 1.6** (*left*) Preload, (*right*) afterload

## Cardiac Output

Cardiac output is the blood volume pumped from the heart in litres per minute. The average male pumps just over five liters a minute while the average female pumps just under five litres per minute at rest. The formula for cardiac output is:

$$CO = SV \times HR$$

With SV being the stroke volume and HR being the heart rate. The stroke volume is calculated by subtracting the end systolic volume (ESV) from the end diastolic volume (EDV):

$$SV = EDV - ESV$$

Various conditions can reduce cardiac output. A reduction in cardiac output may mean that insufficient blood and oxygen is available to perfuse the internal organs. Blood pressure is also dependent on cardiac output.

## Blood Pressure

Is the pressure of the blood against the arterial walls, and is usually measured in millimeters of mercury (mmHg). The top number represents the systolic pressure, with the bottom number representing the diastolic pressure. Blood pressure varies amongst individuals and is different throughout the course of the day. High blood pressure is referred to as hypertension whereas low blood pressure is referred to as hypotension. Classifications of blood pressure levels can be seen in Table 1.1.

It is recommended that blood pressure be taken manually in patients with any irregularity in pulse. Automated devices for blood pressure measurement may have poorer accuracy levels if the pulse is variable, as seen in patients with atrial fibrillation. It is also important to use the appropriately sized blood pressure cuff when taking a patients blood pressure.

Blood pressure is determined by multiplying the cardiac output by the systemic vascular resistance (SVR), which is the total resistance to blood flow from the vasculature in the whole body. Sometimes SVR is referred to as total peripheral resistance.

$$BP = CO \times SVR$$

**Table 1.1** Blood pressure classifications

| Category | Systolic BP (mmHg) | Diastolic BP (mmHg) |
| --- | --- | --- |
| **Hypotension** | <90 | <60 |
| **Normal/optimal blood pressure** | | |
| Optimal | <120 | <80 |
| Normal | <130 | <85 |
| High normal | 130–139 | 85–89 |
| **Hypertension** | | |
| Grade 1 (mild) | 140–159 | 90–99 |
| Grade 2 (moderate) | 160–179 | 100–109 |
| Grade 3 (severe) | ≥180 | ≥110 |

Therefore a reduction in cardiac output also has the effect of reducing blood pressure. An average blood pressure taken during the period of a cardiac cycle, termed the mean arterial pressure (MAP) can be determined by multiplying the cardiac output with the systemic vascular resistance and adding the central venous pressure.

$$MAP = (CO \times SVR) + CVP$$

For clinical purposes the MAP can be approximated as follows:

$$MAP \approx dia + \frac{(sys - dia)}{3}$$

(dia=diastolic pressure, sys=systolic pressure)

If the MAP is <60 mmHg, blood pressure is generally insufficient to perfuse the organs. Some electronic observation machines that record blood pressure may also display the mean arterial pressure. An understanding of the relationship between cardiac output, blood pressure and the effect they have on providing sufficient blood/oxygen to the organs of the body provides a basis for understanding the potential problems arising from any reduction in cardiac output due to pathology.

## Electrophysiology

When the heart is functioning correctly, mechanical aspects of the heart are activated by the heart's electrical system at regular intervals. Action potentials generated in the cardiac conduction system cause proteins to contract in contractile cells, leading to mechanical activation of the heart. The cells of the cardiac conduction system are imbued with the ability to spontaneously depolarize. This quality is referred to as automaticity. Figure 1.7 displays the cardiac conduction system.

The atria and ventricles are electrically isolated from each other in the healthy heart. This means that electrical impulses can only pass between atria and ventricles via the specialized conduction pathways. The hearts primary pacemaker is the sino-atrial node (SAN), located in the right atrium. The SAN is composed of self-excitatory cells that discharge electrical impulses at a rate of between 60 and 100 beats per minute (BPM) in a typical person. The determination of the heartbeat by the sinoatrial node is where the term sinus rhythm derives, meaning a rhythm originating from the sinoatrial node. After firing of the SAN the impulse travels to both atria causing the atria to depolarize; this is followed by physical atrial contraction. The impulse then passes through the atrioventricular (AV) node, down the bundle of His and into the left and right bundle branches and finally terminating in the purkinje fibres. The left bundle branch is more complex than the right and has an anterior and posterior fascicle. Following this the ventricles then also depolarize and contract.

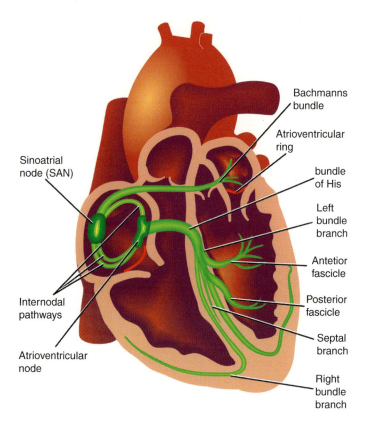

**Fig. 1.7**  The cardiac conduction system

If any problems with the conduction system occur preventing primary pacemaker generation of impulses then other parts of the conduction system are capable of taking over as the dominant cardiac pacemaker. The lower down the conduction system the primary pacemaker is located, the slower the heart rate. The heart rates related to the location of the primary pacemaker can be seen in Table 1.2.

## *Understanding Depolarization and Repolarization*

Depolarization is a process where a resting cell changes from being predominantly negatively charged to positively charged. Repolarization is the reverse of this process with the cell returning to its resting state and predominantly negative charge (Fig. 1.8). The process of depolarization is accomplished by the influx of positively charged extracellular ions into the cell resulting in an action potential (Fig. 1.9). The action potential has various phases (0–4).

**Table 1.2**  Heart rate based on location of primary cardiac pacemaker

| Location of dominant pacemaker in the conduction system | Heart rate (BPM) |
| --- | --- |
| Sinoatrial node | 60–100 |
| Atrioventricular node | 45–60 |
| Purkinje fibres | 15–30 |

**Fig. 1.8**  Depolarization and repolarization

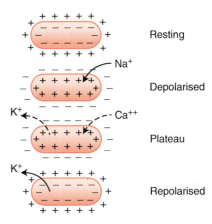

**Fig. 1.9**  Cardiomyocyte action potential

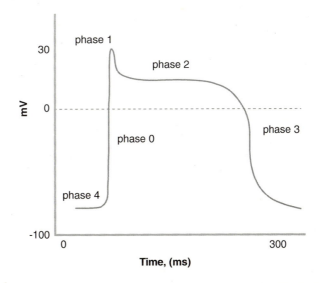

## Phase 0
Represents the rapid depolarisation effect. Phase 0 is triggered when the cell membrane reaches its threshold (around −70 mV). Rapid entry of sodium (Na⁺) occurs.

## Phase 1
Represents the rapid repolarization effect. Flow of sodium ceases as the fast sodium channels close. Potassium continues to leave the cell. As the positive charge of the cellular membrane decreases.

**Phase 2**

Represents a plateau as repolarisation continues but at a slower steady rate. Calcium ($ca^{2+}$) enters the cell causing the release of stored intracellular calcium. The straighterline (seen in phase 2 in Fig. 1.9) is caused by potassium leaving, which causes the charge to become more negative. At the same time calcium causes the charge to become more positive. They in effect cancel each other out to a degree keeping the line relatively straight.

**Phase 3**

Represents the end of the repolarisation phase. The membrane potential returns to its resting state and the inside of the cell starts to become more negative as more potassium is leaving the cell; than calcium is entering causing the membrane potential to become more negative.

**Phase 4**

This represents the gap between one action potential and another. During this time the inside of the cell is more negatively charged. Excess levels of sodium are transported out of the cell with potassium being transported back into the cell.

## Absolute and Relative Refractory Periods

There is a point after initiation of an action potential at which cardiac cells are unable to initiate another action potential no matter how powerful the stimulus is. This is termed the absolute refractory period. The relative refractory period however can transmit impulses but with a delay.

This can be evidenced in AV nodal blocks where impulses arriving at the AV node in the absolute refractory period are not transmitted to the ventricles at all. The earlier the impulse arrives during the relative refractory period the longer it will take to get to the ventricles. AV nodal blocks are discussed in more detail in Chap. 5.

## The Conduction System Related to the Electrocardiogram

The ECG waveform is made up of various waves, intervals and segments representing a single heartbeat (Fig. 1.10).

Understanding of the depolarization and repolarization of the heart and it's relationship to the ECG waveform is necessary to understand the relationship between the electrical and mechanical systems of the heart in a normal person.

The P wave on the ECG represents depolarisation of the right and left atria (Fig. 1.11a). The atria then repolarize as the ventricles begin to depolarize from the apex of the heart upwards leading to the QRS complex on the ECG (Fig. 1.11b, c). Atrial repolarization is not normally visible on the ECG as it is masked by the QRS

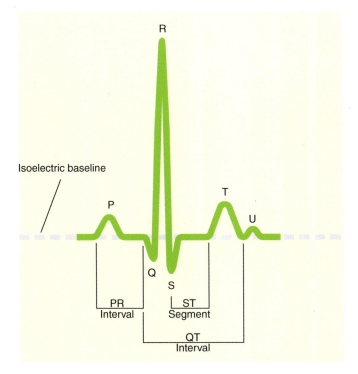

**Fig. 1.10** The ECG waveform

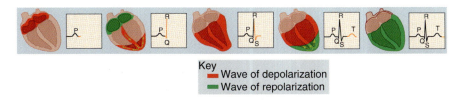

Key
Wave of depolarization
Wave of repolarization

**Fig. 1.11** Conduction system and relationship to the electrocardiogram

complex. The ventricles then begin to repolarize from the bottom of the heart upwards, represented on the ECG by the T wave (Fig. 1.11d, e).

## Summary of Key Points

- The heart has both electrical and mechanical elements
- The sinoatrial node is the dominant pacemaker of the heart
- Any reduction in cardiac output can reduce the amount of blood and oxygen available to the organs of the body
- The circulatory system has two main parts, systemic circulation providing blood to the majority of the body and pulmonary circulation moving blood from lungs to the heart and back again

- In healthy people the electrical system corresponds to mechanical activation of the heart

## Quiz

Q1. The dominant pacemaker of the heart in a healthy person is

 (A)  The atrioventricular node
 (B)  The sinoatrial node
 (C)  The purkinje fibres

Q2. The absolute refractory period is

 (A)  Cellular inability to initiate another action potential no matter how power-ful the stimulus
 (B)  Some impulses can get through, they are just slower
 (C)  Depolarization of the right bundle branch

Q3. The pericardium is

 (A)  A collection of cardiomyocytes capable of spontaneous depolarization
 (B)  The top left chamber of the heart
 (C)  A fibrous sac that surrounds and protects the hearts

Q4. Atrial repolarization is not usually see on the surface ECG

 (A)  True
 (B)  False

Q5. Hypotension refers to

 (A)  Higher than normal blood pressure
 (B)  Lower than normal blood pressure
 (C)  Normal blood pressure

Q6. The lower down the conduction system the primary pacemaker is located the slower the heart rate

 (A)  True
 (B)  False

Q7. For mean arterial blood pressure to adequately perfuse the organs it should be

 (A)  >40 mmHg
 (B)  >60 mmHg
 (C)  >10 mmHg

Q8. The P wave on the ECG represents

    (A) Depolarization of the right and left ventricle
    (B) Repolarization of the right and left atrium
    (C) Depolarization of the right and left atrium

Answers: Q1＝B, Q2＝A, Q3＝C, Q4＝A, Q5＝B, Q6＝A, Q7＝B, Q8＝C

# Chapter 2
# ECG Interpretation

**Keywords** Waveforms • Intervals • Segments • Artefact • Calibration • Rate • Rhythm

## Background

Interpreting the ECG is a task that requires an underpinning knowledge of the way the ECG is organised, what is being displayed and what the normal ranges and values of the various waveforms, intervals and segments should be. In addition to this initial knowledge base practitioners should spend as much time as they can looking at real ECGs in context, and preferably discussing these findings with more experienced colleagues. Like learning to play the piano or developing foreign language proficiency it requires many hours of practice built on top of the basic knowledge gained from books, lectures and other sources.

There are many ways to interpret an ECG. The authors recommend using a systematic approach that includes the following aspects:

- Basic quality control checks
- Rhythm determination
- Rate calculation
- Examination of the morphology and duration of the various waves, intervals and segments
- Determining of the QRS axis
- Scanning for any additional features or abnormalities

We begin by looking at how the ECG is organised on the paper and in leads and move on to look at the normal values for the various components of the ECG waveform, including different methods of calculating the rate and determining the rhythm.

© Springer-Verlag London 2015
A. Davies, A. Scott, *Starting to Read ECGs: A Comprehensive Guide
to Theory and Practice*, DOI 10.1007/978-1-4471-4965-1_2

## ECG Paper

12-lead ECGs are usually displayed on special gridded paper (Fig. 2.1). The 12 leads I, II, III, aVR, aVL, aVF and $V_1$–$V_6$ are displayed on the paper under their respective headings. The limb leads are found on the left hand side and the chest leads V/C 1–6 on the right. The leads are separated by lead divider markers which resemble an elongated punctuation colon (:). The gridded area of the paper is split into larger boxes with smaller boxes inside them. Each large box measures 5 mm² (containing 25 smaller 1 mm² boxes). Time is measured along the x-axis (horizontal) in seconds. Each large box represents 0.2 s of time, with each smaller box measuring 0.04 s. Each lead represents around 3 s of time. Most 12-lead ECGs also include a rhythm strip, shown below the other leads. This strip is one of the existing leads displayed above, shown for around 12 s, usually lead II or $V_1$. This allows interpreters to look for patterns and features that might not otherwise be visible in shorter time periods. Some ECGs have more than one rhythm strip included. The y-axis (vertical) represents the amplitude of the ECG waveforms, measured in millivolts. One large square represents 0.5 mV, with a small square measuring 0.1 mV.

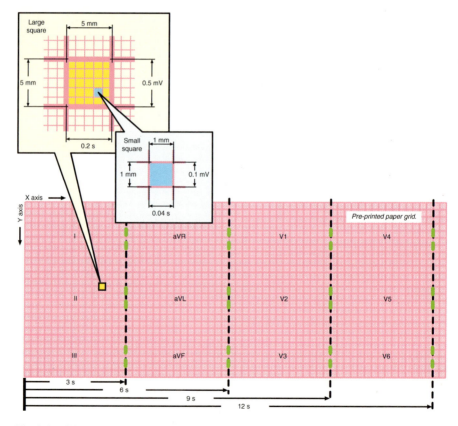

**Fig. 2.1** ECG paper details

# Basic Checks

There are several details that should be checked prior to analysing the waveforms and formulating an interpretation. These checks include:

- Ensuring the ECG is free from artifact and recorded at sufficient quality to enable a subsequent interpretation.
- Checking R wave progression in the chest leads and the deflection of lead aVR
- Checking the calibration markers/calibration signal boxes to ensure the ECG is recorded using the standard settings.

# Artefact

Is any artificial disturbance that negatively impacts on the quality of the ECG. There are many forms of interference that can affect the quality. There are however several types of commonly encountered interference that can be easily recognised and prevented or reduced in most cases. Table 2.1 shows the most common forms of interference, including possible causes and solutions.

# Calibration

Standard ECGs in the UK, USA and many other parts of the world are recorded at a speed of 25 mm/s and a voltage of 10 mm/mV. This is usually displayed on the ECG somewhere (often at the bottom). This information is also displayed graphically in the form of calibration markers, sometimes called calibration signal boxes. These markers look like rectangles (Fig. 2.2) and are usually seen on the left hand side of the ECG preceding the leads.

When the ECG is set up to record at the standard 25 mm/s and 10 mm/mV, the calibration markers should measure 1 cm in height (2 large boxes) by 0.5 cm in width (1 large box). The authors recommend that practitioners recording and interpreting ECGs always check that the ECG was recorded in the standard calibration before attempting interpretation. Speed and amplitude settings can be altered on most ECG machines, it is therefore possible that someone may either deliberately or accidentally alter these settings. If the recording speed was altered to 50 mm/s, it would have the effect of elongating the waveforms, and can make it appear that the patient has an extremely low heart rate and a long QT interval, even though their other observations could otherwise be normal. Sometimes altering these settings is done deliberately. A patient may have a very rapid heart rate making it difficult to see P waves. This can sometimes be overcome by changing the recording speed and elongating the waveforms to see features that would otherwise be missed. Figure 2.3 shows a standard calibration marker and one that is set to 50 mm/s. As shown in the image the second marker is twice as wide as normal, encompassing two large boxes.

**Table 2.1** Common forms of artifact with possible causes and solutions

| Muscle/Somatic tremor | Baseline wander | 60-cycle/AC mains interference |
|---|---|---|
| | | |
| **Cause:** Usually caused by patients moving during a recording. | **Cause:** May be caused by movement of the ECG cables, perspiration or respiratory swing seen in some diseases, such as COPD. | **Cause:** Improper grounding of electrical equipment causing interference or a fractured wire within an ECG cable. |
| **Possible solution(s):** | **Possible solution(s):** | **Possible solution(s):** |
| Ask the patient to remain still during recording. If caused by shivering, ensure patient warm before attempting recording. | Ensure cables are not dangling over the edge of the bed or allowed to move during recording. | Remove the equipment/electrical device causing the interference. In the case of medical equipment turn off any non-essential devices that may be causing the interference. |
| In the case of pathological tremor such as Parkinson's disease, patients can be asked to place their arms under their legs. Modified lead positions can also be used to reduce interference (i.e. shoulders and upper legs). | Cleanse the skin with alcohol wipes to remove oils, debris and perspiration (check for patient sensitivity or religious objections first). Alternatively soap and water may be used. | Ensure patients own electrical equipment is checked by appropriately trained personnel. This is also often carried out for safety reasons. |
| | Ask patient to hold breath if possible, alternatively record ECG in a more upright position (remember to document this on the ECG i.e. ECG recorded in sitting position). | If the fault is not caused by other electrical equipment the ECG machine should be tested and evaluated by the relevant department/personnel. |

**Fig. 2.2** A calibration marker

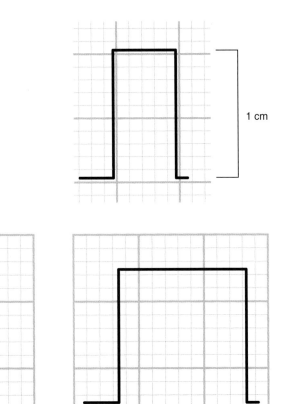

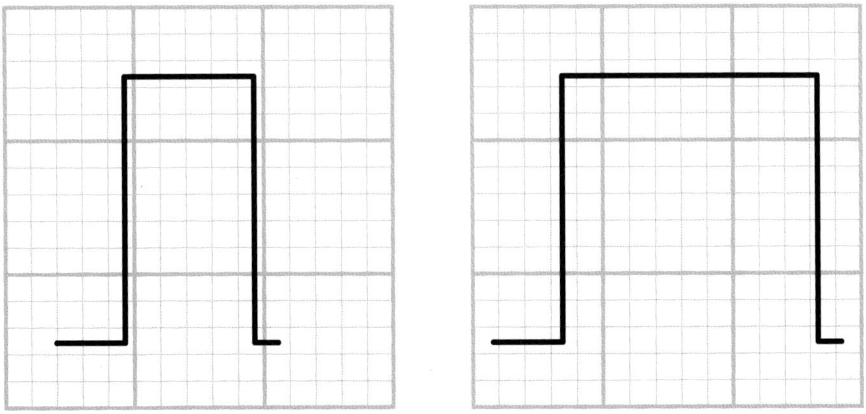

1 cm

**Fig. 2.3** Calibration markers showing differences in recording speeds. 25 mm/s (*left*), 50 mm/s (*right*)

Similar changes can be made to the amplitude of the ECG. Certain conditions, such as left ventricular hypertrophy can cause the height/depth of the waveforms to be very large and they may overlap each other, making the ECG difficult to view. In these cases some practitioners may request the ECG is recorded at half normal voltage. Conversely if a normal ECG is viewed at half voltage the waveforms can appear very small, which can lead to a false interpretation, as it can display false features of conditions like pericardial effusion, which features small voltage deflections. Figure 2.4 shows a calibration marker at half voltage.

Some machines will also allow the voltage to be reduced just for the limb or chest leads, leaving the other leads at normal voltage. This is represented by a calibration marker with a step in it. If the step is on the left it represents a reduction in the limb lead voltage only, whereas a step on the right hand side represents a reduction in the voltage of the chest leads only (Fig. 2.5).

Finally the voltage can be decreased and the recording speed changed simultaneously. This is represented by a small and wide calibration marker (5 mm in height

**Fig. 2.4** Calibration marker
showing ½ voltage (5 mm/
mV)

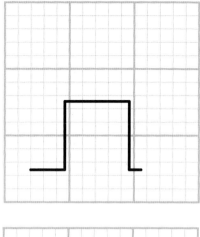

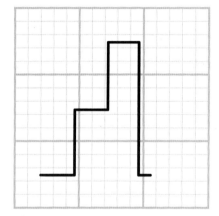

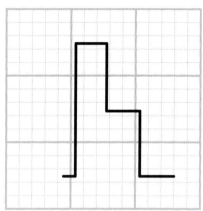

**Fig. 2.5** Reduced limb lead voltage only (*left*), reduced chest lead voltage only (*right*)

and 10 mm in width). Practitioners should be familiar with both normal and adjusted calibration markers, what they represent and what impact changing these settings may have on the interpretation of the ECG. Even though the calibration markers will reflect any changes it is still good practice to document on the ECG any changes to the normal settings made when recording to draw other practitioners attention to these changes explicitly.

## R Wave Progression/Lead aVR

R wave progression refers to the deflection changes that occur in the chest leads ($V_1$–$V_6$) as they move from a predominantly negative to a predominantly positive defection (Fig. 2.6.).

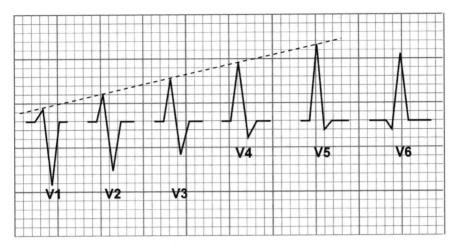

**Fig. 2.6** Normal R wave progression in leads V₁ to V₆

If there are any sudden changes in deflection it is possible that one or more of the chest leads have been placed in the wrong position.

Incorrect lead placement in the limb leads can be identified by a positively deflected lead aVR, especially if the patients previous ECG(s) have a negatively deflected aVR. Lead aVR is nearly always negatively deflected. If it is positive the limb leads may have been applied the wrong way around. This can mimic a condition called dextrocardia, where heart is situated on the right hand side of the chest as oppose to the left. With dextrocardia there is often right axis deviation, positively deflected complexes in lead aVR, negatively deflected complexes in lead I and an absence of R wave progression in the precordial leads. The principle difference between true and technical dextrocardia is that in the later there are no changes seen in the precordial leads.

Basic quality control checks should be carried out by the recorder of the ECG whilst the leads are still in situ. This makes it easier to identify issues such as incorrect lead placement, identification of artifact and any issues with recording settings. Not only is it easier to correct problems at this stage before interpretation is attempted but it also reduces the potential for subsequent interpretation errors.

## Determine the Rhythm

The normal heart rhythm is very rarely exactly regular. The human heart rate has a fractal quality. A fractal is a mathematical term to describe patterns that look similar at progressively smaller scales. Other examples from nature include snowflakes and fern leaves. If you were to zoom in on a snowflake again and again the pattern you

**Fig. 2.7**  Sierpinski's triangle

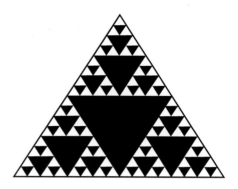

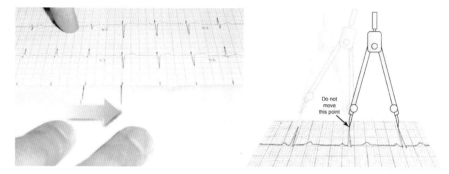

**Fig. 2.8**  The paper method (*left*), caliper method (*right*)

would see would resemble the larger pattern. An example of this self similarity can be seen in Fig. 2.7. The Sierpinski's triangle or gasket as it is sometimes referred is a basic example of self similar sets.

The heart rate itself has a fractal variance making it ever so slightly variable. This is extremely important because if this was not the case the stress on the heart muscle each beat would occur at exactly the same point. This slight variance allows wear and tear of the heart to be dramatically reduced.

For pragmatic clinical purposes however rhythms tend to be defined as either regular or irregular. There are a couple of practical ways rhythms can be checked for irregularity. One of the easiest is to take a piece of paper and place it just under the tip of the R waves on the rhythm strip. Next mark a line directly under two consecutive R waves on the piece of paper. Now move the paper along the rhythm strip and check that the two lines on the paper line up with the preceding R waves (Fig. 2.8). Some practitioners do this with a set of calipers (like a compass for drawing circles but with two needles). The calipers are set to mark the distance between two consecutive R waves then swung between the preceding ones (Fig. 2.8).

When checking the rhythm practitioners should consider the following; is the rhythm regular or irregular? if irregular is there a pattern to the irregularity or not? and are PQRST waves present for each beat?

## Sinus Arrhythmia

Is a normal variation that produces an irregularity in the heart rate. This is caused by the heart rate increasing as the individual breaths in and slowing down when they breath out. Sinus arrhythmia does not cause any symptoms and PQRST waves are all present. Sinus arrhythmia is discussed in more detail in Chap. 6.

## Rate Calculation

The normal adult heart rate is between 60 and 100 BPM. When lying still in bed the normal rate is between 60 and 80 BPM. Normal childrens heart rates can be much higher than adults, for more information on children see Chap. 9, which discusses the pediatric ECG in more detail. With adults anything below 60 BPM is classified as a bradycardia. Anything above 100 BPM is defined as a tachycardia (Table 2.2). Although the ECG can be used to determine the heart rate, a lot of useful information can also be determined from manual palpation of the patients pulse. To feel a pulse slight compression should be made to an artery located against a bone. The common pulse points are shown in Fig. 2.9. Manual inspection of the pulse should not be underestimated. For example; pulseless electrical activity (PEA) is an arrest rhythm where electrical activity is present on the ECG, because the conduction system is working normally, however there is no effective mechanical pumping action taking place and no cardiac output.

There are several different methods for determining the heart rate on the ECG. These calculations vary in accuracy and complexity. Some of the methods only work when the heart rate is regular. Several of these methods are described here in the hope that the reader will select the one(s) that are of the most use to their individual circumstances, and that they will develop an awareness of the existence of other methods. The same ECG is used to demonstrate the different methods.

### *Automated Rate Determination*

Most modern ECG machines have an automated computerised set of measurements and interpretation statements. These measures often include the various intervals and durations. They usually also include the heart rate, seen in Fig. 2.10 as **Vent rate: 59 BPM**. This states the ventricular rate is 59 beats per minute.

**Table 2.2** Heart rate classifications

| Bradycardia | <60 BPM |
|---|---|
| Normocardia | 60–100 BPM |
| Tachycardia | >100 BPM |

**Fig. 2.9** Palpable pulse points

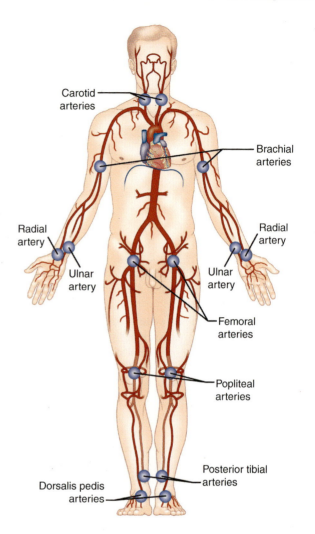

Carotid arteries

Brachial arteries

Radial artery

Ulnar artery

Radial artery

Ulnar artery

Femoral arteries

Popliteal arteries

Posterior tibial arteries

Dorsalis pedis arteries

9-Mar-2012 21:02:05

| | | |
|---|---|---|
| Vent rate: | 59 BPM | SINUS RHYTHM |
| PR int: | 196 MS | NORMAL ECG |
| QRS dur: | 93 MS | |
| QT/QTc: | 428/426 MS | UNCONFIRMED REPORT |
| P-R-T axes: | 49  35  14 | |
| Avg RR: | 1016 MS | |
| QTcB: | 424 MS | |
| QTcF: | 425 MS | |

**Fig. 2.10** Automated ECG measures and interpretation

There are several problems with relying on the automated heart rate measurement on an ECG. On some ECGs the atrial and ventricular rate may be different, many machines i.e. Fig. 2.10 will not show the atrial rate, so it would be potentially necessary for the practitioner to work the atrial rate out manually. Also machines can make mistakes and older machines may not display this information at all. In addition it is important that practitioners are able to work out these measurements independently and understand how they are derived for a more complete understanding of the ECG.

## The 1,500 Method

This method only works on an ECG with a regular rhythm. Count the number of small squares between the center points of two consecutive R waves. Next divide 1,500 by this number. This works because 1,500 small squares is equal to 60 s of time ($1,500 \times 0.04 = 60$). An example of this can be seen in Fig. 2.11.

This example, taken from the same ECG that the automated ECG data is from shows there are 25 small squares between two consecutive R waves on the rhythm strip.

$1,500 \div 25 = 60$ BPM. This is very close to the computerised measure that reports the rate as 59 BPM.

## The 300 Method

The 300 method is less accurate than the 1,500 method but follows the same idea. If 1,500 small boxes is equivalent to a minute, then 300 large squares is also equivalent to a minute, as each large square contains five smaller squares ($1,500 \div 5 = 300$). In this example we can see that there are five large squares between two consecutive R waves (Fig. 2.12). So $300 \div 5 = 60$.

Again this method only works with regular rhythms, and works best when R waves fall on the edges of large squares, as in this example.

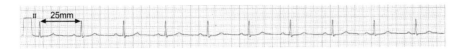

**Fig. 2.11** Taking the same point between two consecutive R waves and counting the small squares

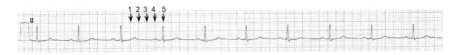

**Fig. 2.12** The 300 method showing that there are five large squares between R waves

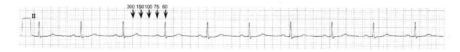

**Fig. 2.13** The number of large boxes between two consecutive R waves

**Table 2.3** The relationship between large box intervals and heart rate

| Number of large squares between two consecutive R waves | Heart rate (BPM) |
|---|---|
| 1 | 300 |
| 2 | 150 |
| 3 | 100 |
| 4 | 75 |
| 5 | 60 |
| 6 | 50 |

## The Sequential Method

This method involves memorising a descending sequence of numbers based on the number of large boxes between two consecutive R waves in a regular rhythm (Fig. 2.13). These numbers are basically derived from the 300 method described previously but rather than working them out, the first six or so are memorised for ease of use.

The relationship between large boxes and R waves can be summarised in Table 2.3. In this example there are five large boxes between two consecutive R waves making the heart rate 60 BPM, which is consistent with the previous methods. This method can be quick and easy provided the practitioner can memorize the sequence. The disadvantage is that it is less accurate, especially when the R waves do not fall on the edge of large squares.

## The 30 Square Method

This method works for both regular and irregular rhythms. A rhythm strip is also required as we need to count 30 large squares. To use this method count any 30 continuous large squares on the rhythm strip (Fig. 2.14). Next count the number of QRS complexes within the 30 large squares (Fig. 2.15). Multiply this number by 10 to determine the BPM. This works because each large square is 0.2 s, so $0.2 \times 30 = 6$. This gives us 6 s of time. This number can then be multiplied by 10 to give us 60 s of time (1 min).

In this example there are six QRS complexes within the 30 large square area. $6 \times 10 = 60$. So the heart rate is 60 BPM.

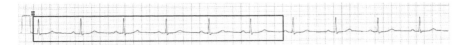

**Fig. 2.14** Count any 30 continuous large squares in the rhythm strip

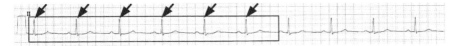

**Fig. 2.15** Count the number of QRS complexes in the 30 large square area

**Table 2.4** Summary of rate calculation methods

| Method name | Method | Rhythm type method works with |
|---|---|---|
| The 1,500 method | $\dfrac{1{,}500}{n}$  n = number of small squares between two consecutive R waves | Regular |
| The 300 method | $\dfrac{300}{n}$  n = number of large squares between two consecutive R waves | Regular |
| The sequential method | Remember the sequence for the number of large squares between two consecutive R waves | Regular |
|  | 300, 150, 100, 75, 60, 50 |  |
| The 30 square method | 1. Count any 30 continuous large squares in the rhythm strip. | Regular/irregular |
|  | 2. Count the number of QRS complexes within the 30 large square area (n) |  |
|  | 3. n × 10 |  |

All the methods described above can also be used to determine the atrial rate as well. Instead of measuring between R waves, measure between the centre points of the P waves. It is possible with certain ECGs that the atrial and ventricular rate may be different and it may be necessary to work out both the atrial and ventricular rate. All of the methods described previously are summarised in Table 2.4.

## Converting Time Between Seconds and Milliseconds

Before examining the various waveforms and intervals it is worth considering how they are measured. Many ECG books describe the length of time on ECGs in

**Table 2.5**  Converting between seconds and milliseconds and vise versa

| Seconds (s) to milliseconds (ms) | Milliseconds (ms) to seconds (s) |
|---|---|
| ms = s × 1,000 | s = ms × 0.001 |

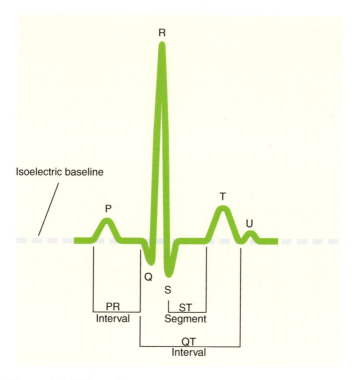

**Fig. 2.16**  The standard ECG waveform as seen in lead II

seconds (s). Many automated ECG measures however tend to display this information in milliseconds (ms). It is recommended that practitioners are comfortable converting between seconds and milliseconds for the purpose of being confident reading these time intervals in their preferred format.

For example the PR interval in the automated measurements in Fig. 2.10 is shown as being 196 ms. To convert this to seconds multiply the milliseconds by 0.001. i.e. 196×0.001 = 0.196 or 0.20 s when rounded to two decimal places. To convert seconds to milliseconds simply multiply the seconds by 1,000 i.e. 0.196×1,000 = 196 ms. This is summarised in Table 2.5.

## The ECG Waveform

Waveforms from lead II are often used in training material because they are positively deflected and contain the principle waves. Figure 2.16 shows an ECG waveform consisting of PQRST and U waves. Each of these waveforms represent an

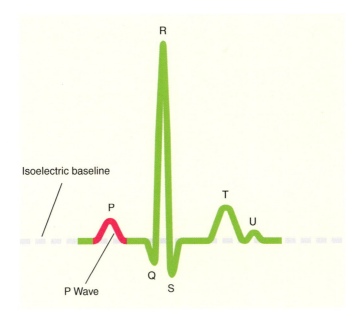

**Fig. 2.17** The P wave

individual heartbeat on the ECG in normal circumstances, more accurately it represents electrical activation of the cardiac conduction system; as electrical activation does not necessarily mean than physical contraction of the heart has taken place. The waves were named P, Q, R, S, T and U instead of A, B, C, etc. because the inventor of the ECG, Willem Einthoven believed that other waves may be discovered before and/or after the initial waves he had described. With this in mind he labeled them from around the middle of the alphabet, to leave space either side for new wave labels. In addition to the waves there are also various intervals and segments that can be measured. It is important to examine each of the waves in turn and the various intervals and segments to make a complete and accurate interpretation.

## P Wave

P waves (Fig. 2.17) should be present before each QRS complex. They should be regular and share the same morphology. Leads II and $V_1$ are good leads to view for P waves. The P wave represents atrial depolarisation. Normal P waves are initiated by electrical activation from the SAN. P waves should be positively deflected in most leads with the exception of lead aVR where deflection is usually negative and $V_1$, where deflection is usually equiphasic. P waves that are inverted or masked by the QRS complex are caused by impulses that activate the atria from below the SAN, such as the His bundle or AV junction. They can also be caused by retrograde

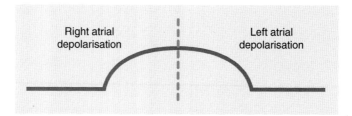

**Fig. 2.18**  P wave showing atrial depolarization

**Fig. 2.19**  The location of the
Ta wave

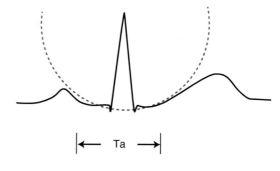

**Fig. 2.20**  Prominent Ta wave

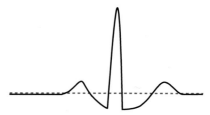

conduction. This is activation of the SAN caused by an impulse travelling back up towards the atria from lower down. The first half of the P wave represents right atrial depolarisation whereas the second half represents depolarisation of the left atria (Fig. 2.18). A normal P wave should not be more than 2.5 mm in width or height.

## Ta Wave

The repolarisation of the atria is represented on the ECG by the Ta wave. This wave is not normally visible on the ECG as it is masked by the QRS complex. The Ta wave is deflected in the opposite direction to it's P wave. Figure 2.19 shows the location of the Ta wave. The wave is better imagined as a curve that sits on top of the waveform. Figure 2.20 shows a prominent Ta wave that is easily recognizable. The Ta wave can also be seen in conjunction with ST elevation or depression.

**Fig. 2.21** The PQ/PR interval

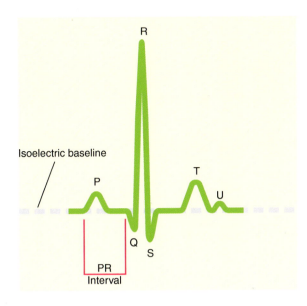

**Table 2.6** Normal PQ/PR interval

| Seconds | Milliseconds | Small squares |
|---|---|---|
| 0.12–0.20 | 120–200 | 3–5 |

## PQ/PR Interval

Measured from the start of the P wave to the start of the QRS complex (Fig. 2.21). The PQ interval can also be referred to as the PR interval if there is no Q wave present. PR/PQ intervals should be consistent in length in different beats and not raised or dipped below the isoelectric baseline. Normal PQ/PR interval duration is shown in Table 2.6. The PQ/PR interval varies in duration due to the heart rate. At a higher rate the interval is shorter and at a lower rate it is longer.

## QRS Complex

The QRS complex (Fig. 2.22) is composed of a Q, R and S waves and represents ventricular depolarisation. The complex looks likes a spike as opposed the dome shaped P wave, this is due to the electrical impulse passing rapidly through the fast conduction pathway. The spike is also much larger than the P wave as the ventricles are much larger than the atria. The complex is measured from the start of the Q wave to the end of the S wave. The normal QRS duration is summarized in Table 2.7.

The QRS complex looks different in different leads. The first negatively deflected wave in the complex is the Q wave, the first positive wave is the R wave and the negative wave after the R wave is the S wave. Not all waves are seen in all leads. The

**Fig. 2.22** The QRS complex

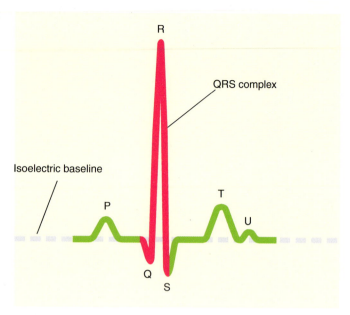

**Table 2.7** Normal QRS complex duration

| Seconds | Milliseconds | Small squares |
| --- | --- | --- |
| 0.06–0.10 | 60–10 | 1.5–2.5 |

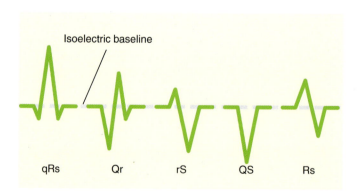

**Fig. 2.23** Variations in QRS appearance

convention is to use a capital letter for a wave with an amplitude >5 mm. When the amplitude is <5 mm a lower case letter is used. Fig. 2.23 demonstrates some of the different appearances of the QRS complex.

## Q Wave

Also called septal Q waves as they represent the depolarisation of the interventricular septum should not be more than 0.04 s (1 small square) in duration. They should also not exceed a 1/3 of the height of the following R wave or be deeper than 2 mm. If Q waves are deep and or wide they may be a pathological finding. Pathological Q waves with no other signs of current myocardial infarction can point towards a previous myocardial infarction. Deeper Q waves are often seen in lead III and do not represent a pathological finding, if they occur in isolation. Q waves are often seen in leads I, aVL, $V_5$ and $V_6$.

## R Wave

The R wave also gets larger from lead $V_1$ to $V_6$. This R wave progression (discussed earlier) can be seen in Fig. 2.6. The amplitude of the R wave is also important. Small amplitude R waves can occur in obese patients or those with pericardial effusion or other myocardial damage. In contrast large R waves can be indicative of an enlarged ventricle. This can be normal in young fit people or a pathological finding related to conditions such as cardiomyopathies. The measure of normal amplitude is dependant on many factors and different assessment criteria exist. Chap. 4 discusses this in more detail.

## QRS Axis

Another useful piece of information that can be determined is the QRS axis. This is the net or overall direction the electrical impulse takes through the ventricles. This can provide additional evidence of certain conditions or help differentiate between others. The subject of QRS axis determination is covered in detail in Chap. 3.

## T Wave

Occurs immediately after the QRS complex and is usually asymmetric in appearance (Fig. 2.24). A normal T wave is deflected in the same direction as the QRS complex (concordant). The height of the T wave can be variable but should not normally exceed the height of the R wave or be flat (level with the isoelectric baseline). Flat, inverted or very tall T waves can all be pathological findings. The T wave

**Fig. 2.24** The T wave

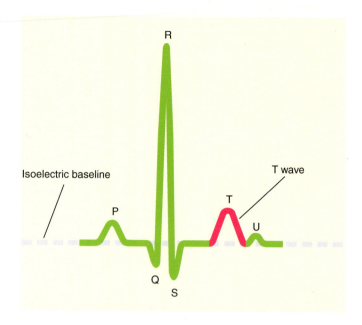

represents the repolarisation of the ventricles. Negatively deflected T waves in leads aVR and $V_1$ are a normal finding. Widespread T wave inversion with no symptoms of pain can also be a normal finding in Afro-Caribbean males.

## U Wave

Not always seen on the ECG, they manifest as a wave proceeding the T wave that is similar in appearance to the P wave but smaller (Fig. 2.25), they are usually concordant with the T wave and best seen in $V_2$ and $V_3$. Although U waves were initially displayed in an ECG trace recorded by the creator of the ECG, Willem Einthoven over a century ago, we still don't know what they actually represent. There are many theories as to the origin of the U wave. Some of the more popular theories are described in Table 2.8.

   U waves can be abnormal if they are prominent or inverted. Prominent U waves are said to be larger than 1 or 2 mm in height. As the heart rate slows down U waves tend to get larger, this makes them easier to see in bradycardic patients. Prominent U waves are also seen in metabolic disturbances such as hypokalaemia. They can also be seen in patients with ventricular hypertrophy or raised intracranial pressure. Certain drugs can also trigger prominent U waves (e.g. Digoxin and some antiarrhythmics). Inverted U waves on the other hand can be a good indicator of various forms of heart disease, including; coronary artery disease, congenital heart disease, cardiomyopathy and valvular heart disease.

**Fig. 2.25** The U
wave

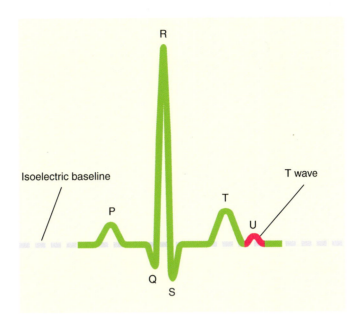

**Table 2.8** Some common theories concerning the
source of U waves

| Repolarisation of the papillary muscle |
| --- |
| Ventricular after potentials |
| Repolarisation of the ventricular septum |
| Delayed repolarisation Purkinje fibres |
| Prolonged repolarisation of midmyocardium cells (M cells) |

## ST Segment

The ST segment (Fig. 2.26) is measured from the end of the S wave to the start of the T wave. This segment marks the delay between the depolarisation and subsequent repolarisation of the ventricle. The J point is the point at which the S wave meets the isoelectric baseline. No additional electrical impulses can pass through the myocardium at this point.

The ST segment should be flat and not elevated above or depressed below the isoelectric baseline. Changes in the ST segment can be indicators of conditions such as acute MI or myocardial ischemia. It is important to examine the ST segment in all leads as pathological changes can occur in some leads and not others. For example an inferior STEMI (ST Elevation Myocardial Infarction) may present with ST elevation in leads II, III and aVF and not be visible in other leads. Myocardial Infarctions, ST elevation and ST depression are discussed in more detail in Chap. 7.

**Fig. 2.26** The ST segment

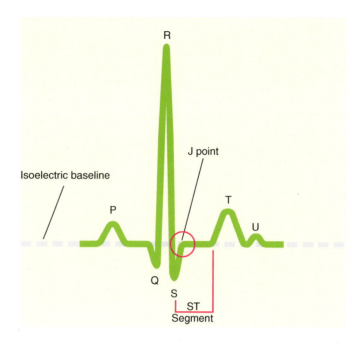

**Table 2.9** Normal QT range

| Seconds | Milliseconds | Small squares ($\approx$) |
|---------|--------------|---------------------------|
| 0.35–0.44 | 350–440 | 8–11 |

## *QT Interval*

The QT interval (Table 2.9) is measured from the start of the QRS complex to the end of the T wave. The interval represents the total time taken from ventricular depolarisation to repolarisation. The QT interval should not be greater than the half the distance between two consecutive R waves.

The QT interval is slightly longer in women than men and also increases with age. Another issue with the QT interval is that it varies according to the heart rate. The higher the heart rate the shorter the QT interval and vise versa. It is said therefore to be inversely proportional to the cardiac rate. To compensate for this there exist a number of formulae that correct for this variance and estimate the QT interval at a rate of 60 BPM. This is termed the corrected QT interval or QTc. Some of the frequently used formulae are displayed in Table 2.10. The most commonly used of these is Bazett's formula, which involves dividing the QT interval in seconds by the square root of the interval between two consecutive R waves in seconds, this is derived in the following way: RR = 60/HR. Although this formula is relatively simple to use and has widespread popularity it often over corrects at high rates and under corrects at lower heart rates. As such using one of the other formulas for patients outside of normocardia may be more accurate.

| Table 2.10 Alternative formulas for calculating the corrected QT interval | Bazett's formula | $QTc = \dfrac{QT}{\sqrt{RR}}$ |
| --- | --- | --- |
| | Fredericia's formula | $QTc = \dfrac{QT}{\sqrt[3]{RR}}$ |
| | Framingham's formula | $QTc = QT + 0.154\ (1 - RR)$ |
| | Hodges formula | $QTc = QT + 1.75\ (heart\ rate - 60)$ |

| Table 2.11 Prolonged QTc in males and females | Gender | Seconds | Milliseconds |
| --- | --- | --- | --- |
| | MALE | 0.44 | 440 |
| | FEMALE | 0.46 | 460 |

**Fig. 2.27** The TP interval

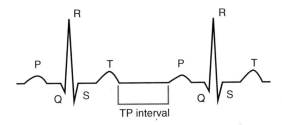

There is no need to correct for the QT interval if the ECG was recorded at 60 BPM. Most ECG machines will calculate the QTc for you but is important to have some understanding of its relevance and the ability to calculate it manually if required. A QTc is considered abnormal if it is too short or too long. Prolonged QTc interval for males and females are shown in Table 2.11. A QTc is considered too short if it is less than 350 ms.

## TP Interval

The TP interval (Fig. 2.27) is the interval between the end of a T wave and the start of the next P wave. This interval is variable and is dependant on the heart rate. Sometime at higher rates the end of one T wave may merge with the subsequent P wave, this is referred to as the TP junction.

## RR Interval

The RR interval is also dependent on the heart rate and is the interval between two consecutive R waves, as seen in Fig. 2.28.

**Fig. 2.28** The RR interval

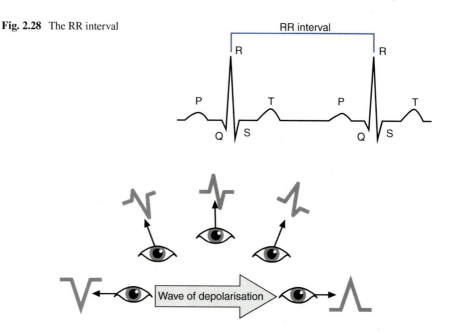

**Fig. 2.29** Deflection

## Why Do the Waveforms Look Different in Different Leads?

The waveforms appear different in various leads due to the direction of the electrical impulse in relation to the lead 'viewing' the impulse.

   As demonstrated by Fig. 2.29, if the impulse travels toward the positive pole of a lead, the wave is positively deflected. If it travels away from the positive pole it is negatively deflected. At various points inbetween it is more or less positively deflected depending on its proximity to the positive pole. If the impulse is at a point exactly between poles it is equiphasically deflected (equally positively and negatively deflected). Leads $V_1$ to $V_6$ look in the horizontal/transverse plane. Leads I, II, III, aVR, aVL and aVF view the heart from the coronal/frontal plane (Fig. 2.30). The areas of the heart viewed by different leads are summarised in Table 2.12.

## Normal Sinus Rhythm

The term normal sinus rhythm is often used to describe an ECG with no abnormalities. It suggests a regular rhythm with a pulse rate of between 60 and 100 BPM. As discussed previously the sinoatrial node is the normal pacemaker of the healthy heart, and in normal circumstances it generates electrical impulses leading to cardiac contraction and rhythmical pulsation in the arteries that is referred to as a pulse.

**Fig. 2.30** ECG
lead views

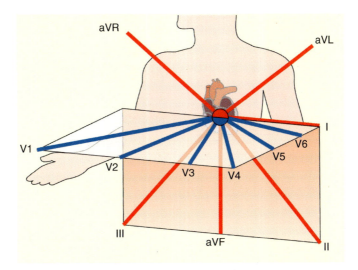

**Table 2.12** Area of heart
viewed by lead

| Lead | Surface/area of heart viewed by lead |
|------|--------------------------------------|
| I | Lateral |
| II | Inferior |
| III | Inferior |
| aVR | Right atrium |
| aVF | Inferior |
| aVL | High lateral |
| $V_1$ | Anterior right ventricle |
| $V_2$ | Anterior right ventricle |
| $V_3$ | Interventricular septum |
| $V_4$ | Apex |
| $V_5$ | Lateral left ventricle |
| $V_6$ | Lateral left ventricle |

The fact that the impulse generating the rhythm originates in the sinoatrial node is where the name sinus rhythm originates. Figure 2.31 shows a 'normal' ECG.

## Summary of Key Points

- It is very important to check the ECG for signs of interference and the settings used to record the ECG as errors can be made subsequently due to these issues. This is especially important if the interpreter is not the person who recorded the ECG.
- The waveforms look different in the different leads, not all parts of the various waves are seen in all leads.

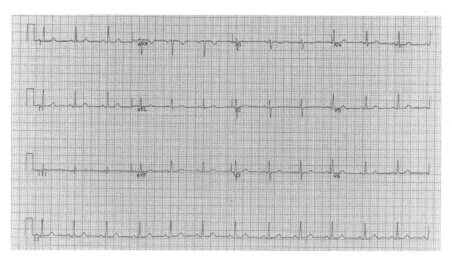

**Fig. 2.31** A 'normal' ECG

- There are many different ways to determine the heart rate that vary in complexity and accuracy. Practitioners should be aware of the different options and use those that are most relevant to their clinical practice.
- There are different formulas that can be used to calculate the QTc. They vary in accuracy and some, such as Bazett's formula work less well at higher and lower rates.
- The exact origin of the U wave is not currently known, although their are many theories currently available.
- Some of the waves and intervals have precise normal values, whereas others are variable and may be influenced by the heart rate, sex or ethnic origin.

## Quiz

Q1. Normocardia (normal heart rate) is.

    (A) < 60 BPM
    (B) 60–100 BPM
    (C) > 100 BPM

Q2. How many milliseconds are there in 3 s?

    (A) 3,000
    (B) 30,000
    (C) 30

Q3. The U wave represents…

    (A) Benign early repolarisation of the right ventricular wall
    (B) Atrial repolarisation
    (C) No one really knows, there are many theories

Q4. All parts of the QRS complex are always visible in all leads.

(A) True
(B) False

Q5. If an impulse travels towards the positive pole of a lead, it is.

(A) Equiphasically deflected
(B) Negatively deflected
(C) Positively deflected

Q6. Bazett's formula is the formula that works the best in any situation.

(A) True
(B) False

Q7. The QTc varies according to gender and age.

(A) True
(B) False

Q8. What are the dimension of calibration markers/signal boxes when the ECG is recorded at the standard 25 mm/s with a voltage of 10 mm/mV.

(A) 1 large box wide by 3 large boxes high (0.5 cm × 1.5 cm)
(B) 2 large boxes wide by 2 large boxes high (1 cm × 1 cm)
(C) 1 large box wide by 2 large boxes high (0.5 cm × 1 cm)

Q9. Would the following ECG be considered to be normal or abnormal?

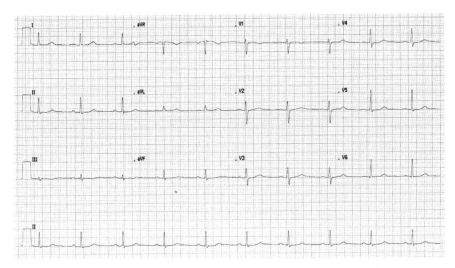

Answers: Q1 = B, Q2 = A, Q3 = C, Q4 = B, Q5 = C, Q6 = B, Q7 = A, Q8 = C, Q9 = normal

# Chapter 3
# Calculating Electrical Axis

**Keywords** Axis • Hexaxial • Vector • Einthoven • Deviation • Bipolar • Unipolar • Deflection • Depolarization

## Background

As electricity is conducted through the ventricles during depolarization, the mean or overall net direction the electricity travels in can be measured. This is often referred to as the cardiac axis or the mean vector (Fig. 3.1). This vector can be calculated and represented in degrees. A vector can be described as a directed quantity of something, in this instance electricity. In most cases when practitioners talk about cardiac axis, they are referring specifically to the mean frontal axis of the QRS complex. It is worth noting however that the axis can be calculated for any part of the waveform.

## How Is This Useful?

Knowing the cardiac axis is useful in two main ways: It helps to confirm certain ECG interpretations and it provides certain supporting evidence for the diagnosis of other conditions as summarised in Table 3.1.

## Normal Axis

The normal cardiac axis is the normal direction electricity takes through the heart. As the apex of the heart is angled to the bottom left and the electrical impulse originates from the top right of the heart, the impulse travels diagonally from the top right to the bottom left in a normal heart (Fig. 3.2).

© Springer-Verlag London 2015
A. Davies, A. Scott, *Starting to Read ECGs: A Comprehensive Guide to Theory and Practice*, DOI 10.1007/978-1-4471-4965-1_3

**Fig. 3.1** The mean vector of depolarisation

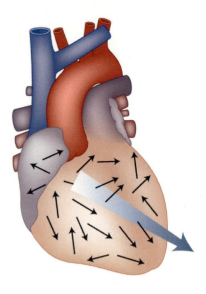

**Table 3.1** Why knowing cardiac axis can be useful

| |
| --- |
| Identification of chamber enlargements such as ventricular hypertrophies |
| Helping to determine if a broad complex tachycardia is ventricular in origin |
| Helping to Identify septal congenital defects |
| Helping to Identify certain conduction defects, such as hemiblocks |
| Assists with the identification of pulmonary embolism |
| Can help identify pre-excitation conduction conditions |

This incidentally is why lead II is one of the most widely used monitoring leads and is often used in textbooks and other examples. Lead II most closely matches the natural direction of the electrical impulse, which runs parallel to lead II. As the wave of depolarisation moves from top right to the bottom left, from a negative to a positive pole it produces the positively deflected classic PQRST waveform (Fig. 3.3).

## Axis Deviation

Simply put axis deviation is a deviation or departure from the expected route of electrical activity. This deviation alters the direction so it is either more to the left or the right of normal. This can be caused by certain conditions, for example MI or hemiblock. It can also be caused by physically moving the heart in the chest (a mechanical shift) for example: pregnancy, ascites or trauma. Different conditions can cause the axis to deviate from the norm. Some examples of these conditions can be seen in Table 3.2.

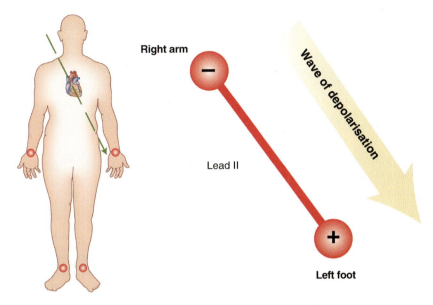

**Fig. 3.2** Direction of depolarisation in a normal heart parallel to lead II

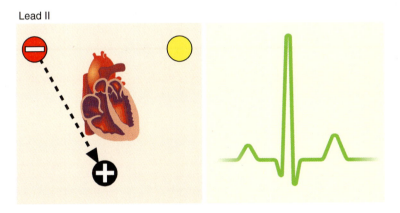

**Fig. 3.3** Lead II and the classic positively deflected waveform seen in that lead

## Categories of Axis Deviation

Normal axis is considered to be between 0° and 90°. Axis deviation can be split into three further sub categories: left, right and extreme right axis deviation (Table 3.3). It is worth mentioning that some experts classify normal cardiac axis to range from −30° to 90° with left axis deviation being −30° to −90°. Extreme right axis is also often referred to by various other names in different texts, including: extreme left axis, no-mans land and right superior axis deviation among others.

**Table 3.2** Causes of left and right axis deviation

| Left axis deviation | Right axis deviation |
|---|---|
| Left bundle branch block (sometimes) | Right bundle branch block (sometimes) |
| Left ventricular hypertrophy | Right ventricular hypertrophy |
| Wolff-Parkinson-White syndrome (sometimes) | Left posterior hemiblock |
| Aortic stenosis | Pulmonary stenosis/hypertension |
| Aging | Emphysema |
| Hyperkalaemia | Lateral wall MI |
| Inferior wall MI | Dextrocardia |
| Mechanical shift | Mechanical shift |
| Normal variation | Normal variation |

**Table 3.3** Axis categorization

| Normal | 0° to 90° or −30° to 90° |
|---|---|
| Left axis deviation | 0° to −90° or −30° to −90° |
| Right axis deviation | 90° to 180° |
| Extreme right axis deviation | −180° to −90° |

# Calculating the Cardiac Axis

There are many different methods that can be used to calculate the cardiac axis. These methods differ in their complexity and accuracy. As such, we present three methods that can be used in clinical settings. Before giving examples of these methods it is worth understanding how the leads work, so that these methods may be easier to understand.

## *Einthoven's Law*

Willem Einthoven, the Dutch physiologist who won the Nobel prize in 1924 for inventing the ECG determined a law that stated:

$$I + (-II) + III = 0$$

Also known as Einthoven's law. It basically means that if you add the waveform amplitudes from the three leads together they cancel each other out and equal zero. The polarity in lead II is switched. Polarity is flow of electrons from one pole to the other (negative to positive). Reversing the polarity changes the direction of the flow of electrons. It is speculated that Einthoven did this because he prefered to view waveforms upright.

To prove that this law works we look in the limb leads (leads I, II and III). We then take away the height of the S wave from the height of the R wave in all three of the leads. Figure 3.4 shows the waveforms in leads I to III. For example the R wave in lead I is positively deflected above the baseline by 5 mm in height, the S wave however is negatively deflected 2 mm below the baseline. Now we take the S wave away from the R wave $5-2=3$. Lead II has a very small R wave just 1 mm in height. The S wave in lead II is 3 mm. $1-3=-2$. Finally the R wave in lead III is just ½ a mm in height (0.5 mm), but has a deep S wave measuring 5.5 mm. $0.5-5.5=-5$

This is summarized in Table 3.4.

As the QRS waveforms can look different in the different leads, it is worth recollecting the variation in appearance of the QRS waveform. This is summarized in Table 3.5.

The values can now be added to the formula. It's worth noting that the sign of the value for lead II is always opposite. For example if the number is negative it becomes positive, alternatively if it is positive it then becomes negative.

$$I+\left(-II\right)+III=0$$
$$\therefore 3+2-5=0$$

As seen in this example $(3+2-5=0)$ the leads all add up to 0. This proves Einthoven's law. These leads form an electrical equilateral triangle, which is termed Einthoven's triangle (Fig. 3.5).

## Bipolar and Unipolar Leads

The original three leads making up Einthoven's triangle are bipolar leads as they have both a positive and negative pole. The original triangle made of equal angles of 60° had wide gaps, which later went onto be filled by unipolar 'V' leads. These V leads took an average of the signal from between the other leads (Fig. 3.6) adding more 'views' of the heart. Unipolar leads have a positive pole located at the recording electrode and a negative pole located at a central terminal. The term unipolar is a little misleading as unipolar leads do have two poles. The difference is in using a central terminal, made up of a composite of other leads as a negative pole, instead of the difference between two leads which were used in the original bipolar leads.

The concept of a central terminal was initially developed by Frank Wilson in the early 1930s and was termed Wilson's central terminal. The disadvantage was that the amplitude of the signals was quite small and so required boosting or augmenting, which was subsequently carried out in the 1940s by Emanuel Goldberger; hence the names aVR, aVF and aVL with the 'a' standing for augmented that were used in Goldberger's central terminal. The precordial 'V' leads $V_1-V_6$ did not require augmenting as the electrodes are placed in close physical proximity to the heart.

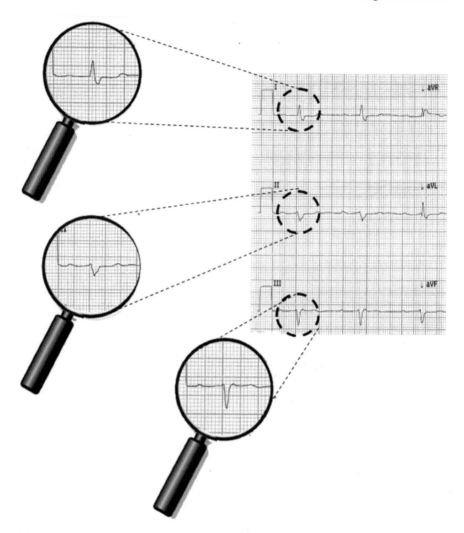

**Fig. 3.4**  Waveforms in leads I to III

**Table 3.4**  R, S and R – S values

| Lead | R wave | S wave | R – S |
|------|--------|--------|-------|
| I    | 5      | −2     | 3     |
| II   | 1      | −3     | −2    |
| III  | 0.5    | −5.5   | −5    |

**Table 3.5** QRS waveform variation

| QRS waveforms |
| --- |
| The first downwards pointing wave in the QRS complex is called the Q wave. |
| The first upward pointing complex is called the R wave. |
| The downward pointing wave following the R wave is called the S wave. |

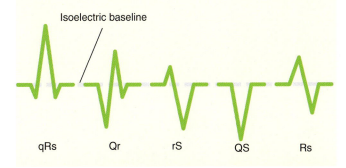

Examples of variation in QRS appearance

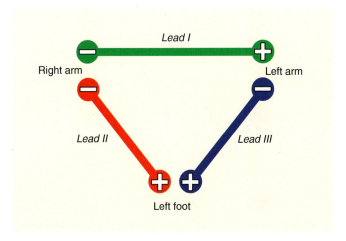

**Fig. 3.5** Einthoven's triangle

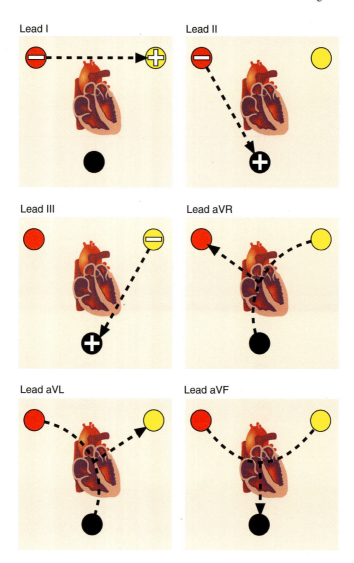

**Fig. 3.6** Augmented 'V' leads derived from original bipolar leads

Three methods of determining the mean frontal QRS axis in clinical practice will now be explored. The complexity and accuracy varies between the methods.

## *Method 1*

In order to better understand how this method works it is worth recapping on waveform deflection. If the wave of depolarisation travels toward the positive pole of a lead, it is positively deflected, in contrast when it moves towards the negative pole it is negatively deflected. If it is at right angles to the lead, it is deflected equiphasically (half up and half down). Anything between these points is deflected biphasically, with the deflection favoring the pole it is closest to. This can be summarized in Fig. 3.7. An example of this in action with lead I can be seen in Table 3.6.

Knowing how the waveform is deflected differently based on the wave of depolarisation relative to the lead allows us to get an idea of the axis by visually inspecting the waveform in a couple of leads. This is one of the easiest but less accurate methods used to determine the QRS axis. Start by looking in leads I and aVF (Table 3.7). If the QRS complexes in these leads are both positively deflected, then axis can be said to be normal. If however the axis in lead I is positive and negative in lead aVF then the axis is left. The opposite (negative lead I, positive lead aVF) indicates right axis.

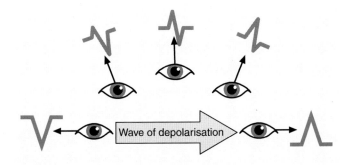

**Fig. 3.7** Deflection

**Table 3.6** Waveform resulting in wave of depolarisation relative to lead I

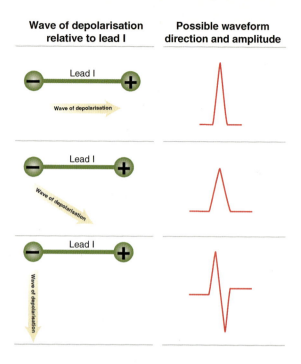

| Wave of depolarisation relative to lead I | Possible waveform direction and amplitude |

**Table 3.7** Quick look method of QRS axis determination

| Lead I (deflection) | Lead aVF (deflection) | AXIS |
|---|---|---|
| ∧ | ∧ | Normal axis |
| ∧ | ∨ | Left axis |
| ∨ | ∧ | Right axis |
| ∨ | ∨ | Extreme right axis |

Finally a negative deflection in both I and aVF indicates extreme right axis deviation. Although this method is relatively easy to remember and use in clinical practice, it lacks precision and makes it difficult to determine borderline cases.

For example, Fig. 3.8 shows positively deflected QRS complexes in lead I and negatively deflected QRS complexes in lead aVF. Using the simple quick look method, we can see that this ECG shows a left axis deviation.

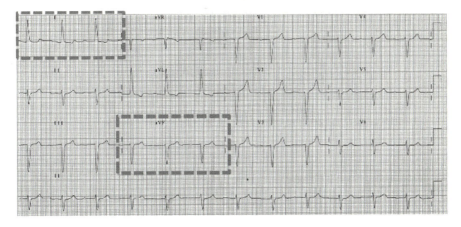

**Fig. 3.8** Left axis deviation

**Fig. 3.9** The hexaxial
reference system

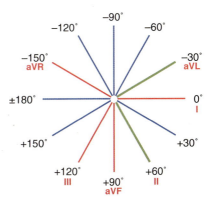

## *Method 2*

This method is more precise and allows the practitioner to quantify the axis in degrees. To use this method one must become familiar with the hexaxial reference system. If you imagine that the leads from Einthoven's triangle are rearranged by moving them inwards until they cross each other. The other leads are then added to the diagram to produce what is known as the hexaxial reference system (Fig. 3.9). At first glance this diagram can seem quite complex and daunting. When starting out with this method, it is worth keeping a copy of the diagram to hand to refer to. In time it becomes so familiar that it can be recreated from memory.

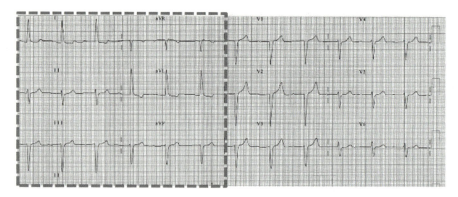

**Fig. 3.10** Leads I, II, III, aVR, aVL and aVF

**Fig. 3.11** Lead aVR and lead III at right angles to each other

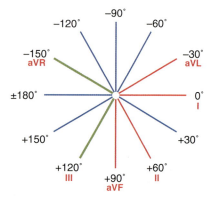

For this method, find the smallest or the most equiphasic lead from among the leads: I, II, III, aVR, aVL and aVF (Fig. 3.10).

In this example the smallest QRS complex is found in lead aVR. Using the hexaxial reference system we find lead aVR and then the lead at right angles (Fig. 3.11). In this case it is lead III.

Now look again at the ECG again and see if the QRS complex in lead III is positively or negatively deflected. In this case it is negatively deflected. Look again at the hexaxial reference system. If the lead was positively deflected we would go the positive pole on the diagram (where the lead name is) as it's negative in this example we go the opposite way (Fig. 3.12). We can see that the axis in this case is −60°. This indicates left axis deviation.

The accuracy of this method can sometimes be further improved. Go back to the original lead on the ECG (the smallest or most equiphasic). Now check to see if the deflection is more positive or negative. If the deflection is more positive we can move 15° closer to the positive pole (subtract 15 from answer), if the deflection is however more negative we can move 15° closer to the negative pole (add 15 to the answer). Finally if the deflection is equiphasic then no further adjustment is possible. In this example the deflection is more negative so we can add 15 to our answer − 60° + 15° = − 45°.

**Fig. 3.12** Axis – 60°

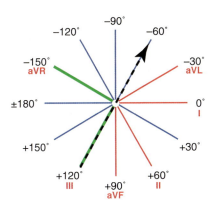

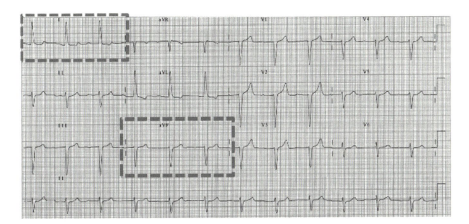

**Fig. 3.13** Leads I and aVF

## *Method 3*

Looking again at lead I and lead aVF (Fig. 3.13).

Work out the net amplitude by subtracting the negative deflection from the positive deflection. In this example we get a positive deflection of +14 mm in lead I and −12 mm in lead aVF. We can plot this on a grid (Fig. 3.14) and then draw lines to see where the points intersect.

We can then draw a line through the point of intersection to determine the QRS axis in degrees (see Fig. 3.15).

In this example we can see the axis shows a left axis deviation of just over 40°.

It is advisable for the practitioner to pick a method that suits their needs and to try to practice that method until they become proficient. Many consider calculating the cardiac axis to be one of the most difficult aspects of ECG interpretation. It can certainly seem that way when first presented with graphs and diagrams showing degrees and numbers. In reality a school child could easily calculate the

**Fig. 3.14** Grid overlaying
the hexaxial reference system

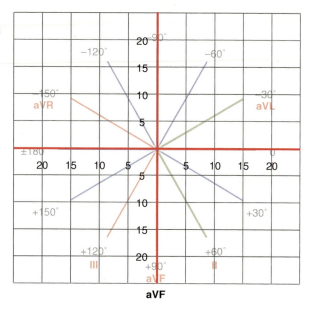

**Fig. 3.15** QRS axis showing
left axis deviation

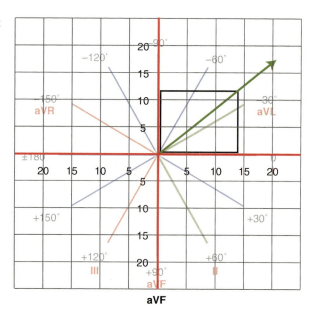

cardiac axis as long as they follow a systematic method. It is more a matter of becoming familiar with your chosen method and practising it frequently with real ECGs.

## Summary of Key Points

- Cardiac axis the mean direction the wave of depolarisation takes through the heart
- There are different methods that can be used to calculate the cardiac axis, these methods vary in complexity and accuracy
- Axis can be determined for each part of the PQRSTU waveform
- Knowing the cardiac axis is useful for providing additional evidence of certain conditions and helping to distinguish others
- Practitioners should choose and practice a method that suits their needs

## Quiz

Q1. If a wave of depolarisation is travelling toward the positive pole of a lead, it will be...

(A) Negatively deflected
(B) Positively deflected
(C) Equiphasically deflected

Q2. Normal cardiac axis is said to be...

(A) $0°$ to $90°$ or $-30°$ to $90°$
(B) $10°$ to $80°$ or $-10°$ to $80°$
(C) $-0°$ to $-90°$ or $-30°$ to $-90°$

Q3. Einthoven's law states that the sum of the three limb leads equals?

(A) 10
(B) −190
(C) 0

Q4. An axis deviation can be caused by a mechanical shift

(A) True
(B) False

Q5. Calculating the cardiac is...

(A) An academic exercise
(B) Of clinical value as it can provide supporting evidence for various conditions
(C) Something you learn just to pass an ECG exam

Q6. The lead that most closely parallels the cardiac axis in a normal heart is...

(A) Lead III
(B) Lead I
(C) Lead II

Work out the axis for the following ECGs using any of the methods above.

**Q7.**

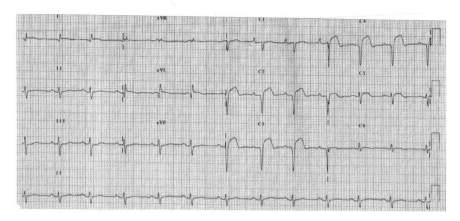

**Q8.**

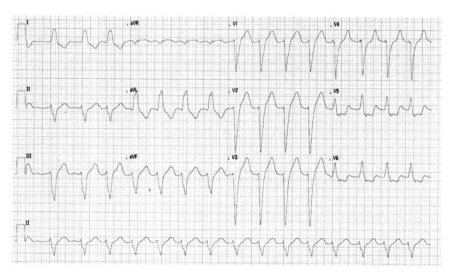

Answers:  Q1 = B,  Q2 = A,  Q3 = C,  Q4 = A,  Q5 = B,  Q6 = C,  Q7 = Normal  axis,
    Q8 = Left axis deviation

# Chapter 4
# Chamber Abnormalities

**Keywords** Hypertrophy • Atrial abnormality • Cardiomyopathy • Heart failure • Voltage criteria • Cardiac resynchronization therapy • Biventricular pacing

## Background

Any physiological changes to the myocardium that cause a chamber to become enlarged or a chamber wall to become thicker than normal can cause ECG changes. There are several mechanisms that cause chamber enlargement and/or thickening to occur, including: hyperplasia, hypertrophy and dilation.

Hyperplasia is the rapid proliferation of cells that can increase the size of the heart. It is also one of the initial stages of tumor development. In contrast hypertrophy is an increase in the size of the cells. This is summarized in Table 4.1. Another cause for the increase in the size of a chamber is caused by dilation of the chamber. This manifests as an increase in the radius of the chamber.

An increase in either pressure or volume can cause enlargement of a hearts chamber (Fig. 4.1). Pressure overload causing hypertrophy is due to the excess pressure required to eject blood from the chamber. This can be the result of systemic hypertension. Volume overload is often caused by regurgitation of blood into the chamber increasing its size by dilation. This is often seen in heart failure and valve regurgitation patients.

An enlargement can occur in any of the main chambers of the heart. The changes in the size of the chambers can often be seen on the ECG. An abnormality in a chamber will show up differently on the ECG depending on which chamber is affected. It is also worth noting that several chambers can be affected in the same patient.

## Atrial Abnormality

The morphology of the P wave gives the practitioner information about the atria.

If one were to draw a line through the center point of a normal P wave, the first half would represent depolarisation of the right atrium, the second half the

© Springer-Verlag London 2015
A. Davies, A. Scott, *Starting to Read ECGs: A Comprehensive Guide
to Theory and Practice*, DOI 10.1007/978-1-4471-4965-1_4

**Table 4.1**  Hyperplasia and hypertrophy

What are hyperplasia and hypertrophy?

**NORMAL CELLS**

**HYPERPLASIA + HYPERTROPHY**

**HYPERPLASIA**        **HYPERTROPHY**

**Hyperplasia**: Cells reproduce rapidly causing the enlargement of an organ or other tissue

**Hypertrophy**: Cells increase in size leading to the enlargement of an organ or tissue.

**Hyperplasia + hypertrophy:** Both of these can occur together (a proliferation of larger cells).

**Fig. 4.1**  Pressure and volume overload

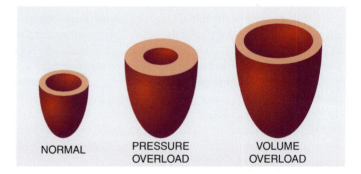

NORMAL        PRESSURE OVERLOAD        VOLUME OVERLOAD

depolarisation of the left atrium (Fig. 4.2). A normal P wave should be no more than 2.5 mm in height and width. The P wave should also be smooth and uniform in appearance. Any change in duration, amplitude or shape indicates the possibility of an abnormality.

## Abnormality or Enlargement?

The terms abnormality and enlargement are often used interchangeably. Since we do not know if these morphological changes are caused by dilation, hypertrophy or an alteration in electrical activation it is more accurate to use the term abnormality than enlargement.

**Fig. 4.2** P wave showing activation of both the left and right atrium

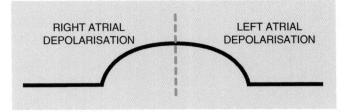

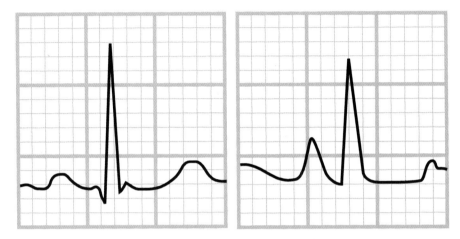

**Fig. 4.3** A normal P wave (*left*), tall peaked P wave with amplitude >2.5 mm (*right*)

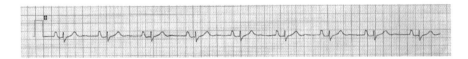

**Fig. 4.4** Tall P waves seen on rhythm strip of ECG (lead II)

## Right Atrial Abnormality

Right atrial abnormality (RAA) is also known as P. pulmonale and is identified on the ECG by a tall, peaked P wave >2.5 mm in amplitude (Figs. 4.3 and 4.4). P waves are often best observed in leads II, III and aVF. The term P. pulmonale derives from the fact that RAA is often seen in patients with pulmonary conditions, such as: pulmonary hypertension, stenosis and embolus.

Another clue can be seen in lead $V_1$. As mentioned previously the first half of the P wave represents right atrial depolarization, the second half, left depolarization. Figure 4.5 shows a normal P wave in lead $V_1$. Both halves of the P wave are fairly equally deflected positively and negatively.

**Fig. 4.5** Normal P wave as seen in lead V$_1$

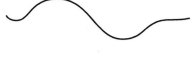

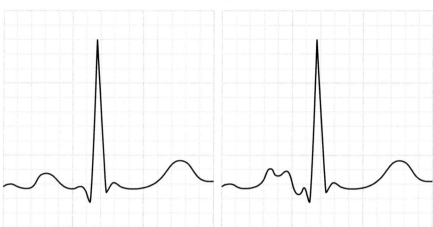

**Fig. 4.6** Normal P wave (*left*), bifid P wave, width >2.5 mm (*right*)

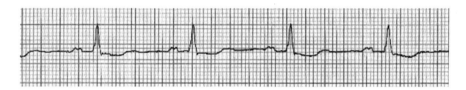

**Fig. 4.7** Bifid ('M' shaped) P waves seen on the rhythm strip of and ECG (lead II)

If there is a RAA present, the first half of the P wave in lead V$_1$ (representing right atrial depolarization) will increase its amplitude by 1.5 mm or more.

## Left Atrial Abnormality

Left atrial abnormality (LAA) also known as P. mitrale as it is often associated with mitral valve disease. LAA is identified on the ECG by bifid (notched) P waves, best seen in leads II and V$_1$. The notching of the P waves represents a letter 'M' in shape (Figs. 4.6 and 4.7).

In lead V$_1$ the second half of the P wave (terminal negative portion) will be negatively deflected by more than 1 mm.

**Table 4.2** Summary of features of atrial abnormalities/enlargements

| Abnormality/enlargement | Lead II | Lead $V_1$ | Features |
|---|---|---|---|
| Right atrial abnormality/enlargement | | | Tall peaked P waves with amplitude >2.5 mm in lead II. First half of the P wave in lead $V_1$ >1.5 mm in amplitude |
| Left atrial abnormality/enlargement | | | Bifid 'M' shaped P waves in lead II. Second half of P wave negatively deflected >1 mm in lead $V_1$. |
| Right/Left atrial abnormality/enlargement | | | Features of both left and right atrial enlargement seen together. Tall, wide bifid P waves. |

## Bilateral Atrial Abnormality

This refers to the presence of both RAA and LAA on the same ECG. Tall and wide notched P waves are present. Table 4.2 summarises the main features of the different types of atrial abnormality.

## Left Ventricular Hypertrophy

One of the primary clues to the presence of left ventricular hypertrophy (LVH) is an increase in QRS voltage on the ECG (Fig. 4.8). This increase is due to the increased muscle mass of the hypertrophied ventricle, which increases the amount of time it takes for electricity pass through the muscle. The presence of large R waves on an ECG should alert the practitioner to the possibility of LVH. LVH is frequently caused by hypertension, cardiomyopathy and aortic regurgitation/stenosis. When documenting findings on the ECG it is better practice to state that voltage criteria for LVH are met, as an echocardiogram would be required to confirm the diagnosis. LVH can also prolong ventricular activation time.

### *Athlete's Heart/Physiological LVH*

Sometimes voltage criteria exists for LVH without ST segment/T wave changes or any other normal signs or symptoms of LVH. This is a normal variant and is often seen in the young, tall thin people and athletes hence the name 'athlete's heart' that is often used to describe this variant (Fig. 4.9). When presented with tall R waves practitioners should also be aware of other potential causes as well as hypertrophy. A summary of these can be seen in Table 4.3.

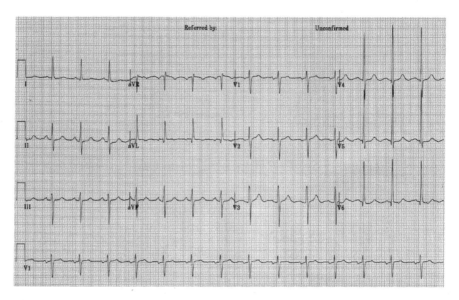

**Fig. 4.8** Voltage criteria for left ventricular hypertrophy

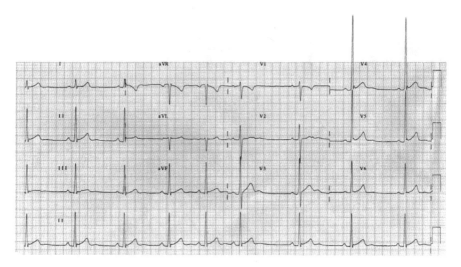

**Fig. 4.9** 'Athletes heart'

## Intrinsicoid Deflection/Ventricular Activation Time (VAT)

The intrinsicoid deflection or ventricular activation time (VAT) is often prolonged in the presence of an intraventricular conduction delay or ventricular hypertrophy. The VAT is measured from the start of the Q wave or R wave to the peak of the R wave (Fig. 4.10). This measure indicates the time it takes for an electrical impulse to reach the hearts surface below the electrode, measured in seconds.

**Table 4.3** Other causes of tall R waves on the ECG

| Other causes of tall R waves |
| --- |
| Incorrect ECG machine calibration |
| Normal variant |
| Right bundle branch block (RBBB) |
| Ventricular rhythms originating in the left ventricle |
| Posterior Myocardial Infarction (MI) |
| Wolff-Parkinson-White syndrome (WPW) |
| Dextrocardia |

**Fig. 4.10** Intrinsicoid deflection/ventricular activation time

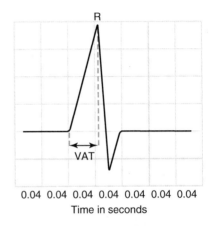

0.04 0.04 0.04 0.04 0.04 0.04 0.04
Time in seconds

**Table 4.4** Summary of VAT normal ranges

| Ventricular activation time (normal ranges) |
| --- |
| Lead $V_1$ |
| **< 0.03 s** |

The normal time in seconds is around 0.02 s in $V_1$ and 0.04 s in leads $V_5$ or $V_6$ (Table 4.4). Any increase means there was a delay in impulse travel time. In the case of ventricular hypertrophy this is caused by the increased time it takes for the impulse to travel through the enlarged chamber.

## Ventricular Hypertrophy Evaluation Methods

There are numerous methods available to help clinicians evaluate ventricular hypertrophy. These methods vary in complexity and precision. The authors would recommend learning the method that is the most appropriate for their clinical role and the one they find the most practical to use and remember. The various scoring systems and criteria are summarised in Tables 4.5, 4.6 and 4.7.

**Table 4.5** The Sokolow-Lyon criteria for LVH

| Sokolow-Lyon criteria for LVH |
| --- |
| S wave in lead $V_1$ + R wave in leads $V_5$ or $V_6 \geq 3.50$ mV (35 mm) |
| **OR** |
| R wave in $V_5/V_6 \geq 2.60$ mV (26 mm) |

**Table 4.6** The Cornell voltage criteria for LVH

| Cornell voltage criteria for LVH | |
| --- | --- |
| Males | R wave in aVL + S wave in $V_3 > 2$ mV (20 mm) |
| Females | R wave in aVL + S wave in $V_3 > 2.8$ mV (28 mm) |

**Table 4.7** The Romhilt-Estes scoring system for LVH (5 = LVH, 4 = probable LVH)

| Romhilt-Estes scoring system for LVH | Points |
| --- | --- |
| An R or S wave in a limb lead $\geq 2$ mV (20 mm) | 3 |
| or S in $V_1$, $V_2$ or $V_3 \geq 3$ mV (30 mm) | |
| or R in $V_4$, $V_5$ or $V_6 \geq 3$ mV (30 mm) | |
| Signs of left ventricular strain: ST-segment/T-wave in opposite direction to QRS complex | |
| Without digoxin | 3 |
| With digoxin | 1 |
| Signs of left atrial enlargement | 3 |
| Left axis deviation $\geq -30°$ | 2 |
| QRS duration $\geq 0.09$ s | 1 |
| Intrinsicoid deflection in $V_5$ or $V_6 \geq 0.05$ s | 1 |

## *Left Ventricular Hypertrophy Evaluation*

The Sokolow-Lyon criteria for LVH is arguably one of the easier to use evaluation methods as it is easier to remember (Table 4.5). If the S wave in $V_1$ is added to the R wave in leads $V_5$ or $V_6$ and if the combined value is 35 mm or more, then voltage criteria for LVH is present. The same is also true if any R waves in $V_5$ or $V_6$ are 26 mm or more.

The Cornell criteria (Table 4.6) works in a similar way to the Sokolow-Lyon criteria but differentiates between males and females. When the R wave in lead aVL is added to the S wave in $V_3$ and the total is greater than 20 mm in men or 28 mm in a woman then voltage criteria for LVH has been met.

The Romhilt-Estes scoring for LVH (Table 4.7) utilizes a scoring system to identify the possibility of LVH and is more involved than the previous two methods. The ECG is examined for various criteria with points awarded for the presence of the various criteria. A total score of 5 = LVH, whereas a score of 4 = probable LVH.

## Right Ventricular Hypertrophy

Right ventricular hypertrophy (RVH) can often be more challenging to identify on the ECG. Tall R waves in $V_1$ should alert the practitioner to the possible presence of RVH (Fig. 4.11). Other clues may also provide supporting evidence. Another

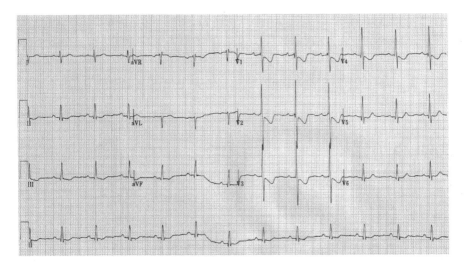

**Fig. 4.11**  voltage criteria for right ventricular hypertrophy

| Table 4.8 The Sokolow-Lyon criteria for RVH | Sokolow-Lyon criteria for RVH |
| --- | --- |
| | R wave in lead $V_1$ + S wave in leads $V_5$ or $V_6 \geq 1.10$ mV (11 mm) |

| Table 4.9 Some common features of RVH (not all of these may be present) | Common features of RVH |
| --- | --- |
| | Right axis deviation |
| | Tall R waves in lead $V_1$ |
| | R wave in $V_1$ + S wave in $V_6 > 1$ mV (10 mm) |
| | Right atrial abnormality |
| | In severe cases associated ST-segment changes, including ST depression and T wave inversion due to 'strain'. |

challenge can be identifying RVH in the presence of a right bundle branch block. In this instance the voltage criteria no longer applies, instead the practitioner should look for additional supporting evidence (Table 4.9) to support their supposition.

## *Right Ventricular Hypertrophy Evaluation*

There are also several different methods for evaluating the presence of right ventricular hypertrophy. Sokolow-Lyon criteria for RVH also exists (Table 4.8). It is also helpful to look common features that provide additional evidence for the presence of RVH. These common features are summarised in Table 4.9.

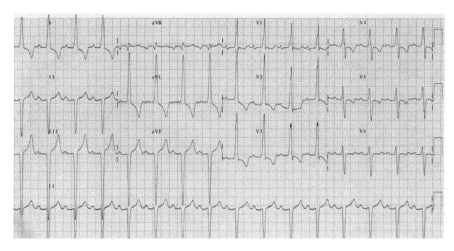

**Fig. 4.12**  Biventricular hypertrophy

## *Biventricular Hypertrophy*

Hypertrophy may occur in both ventricles. Biventricular hypertrophy can be challenging to identify as the hypertrophy in the two ventricles may cancel each other out to some degree on the ECG causing the ECG to look more or less normal. Voltage criteria for LVH in the limb leads coupled with tall R waves in $V_1$ can provide a clue to the presence of biventricular hypertrophy. Biventricular hypertrophy can be seen in Fig. 4.12.

## Cardiomyopathies

A cardiomyopathy is a deterioration of the myocardium that can eventually progress to heart failure. Patients with cardiomyopathy are at increased risk of sudden cardiac death and arrhythmias. There are several different types of cardiomyopathy:

• Dilated cardiomyopathy (DCM)
• Hypertrophic cardiomyopathy (HOCM/HCM)
• Takotsubo cardiomyopathy
• Arrhythmogenic right ventricular cardiomyopathy/Arrhythmogenic right ventricular dysplasia (ARVC/ARVD)

## *Dilated Cardiomyopathy (DCM)*

This is the most common type of cardiomyopathy and affects around 40 in every 100,000 people in the western world. It is also a major reason for cardiac transplantation. The main characteristics include dilation of the left ventricle (Fig. 4.13) and

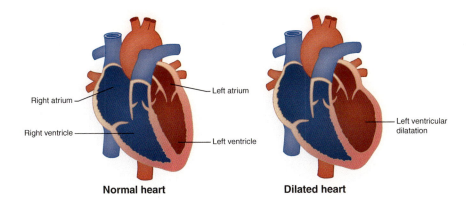

**Fig. 4.13** Normal heart (*left*), dilated heart (*right*)

LV systolic dysfunction. The dilation can also affect the mitral and tricuspid valves leading to regurgitation. Pulmonary congestion occurs due the impaired function of the left ventricle and reduced cardiac output. This can then progress to affect systemic circulation. In many cases right ventricular dilation/dysfunction is also present.

The primary cause of LV dysfunction is a myocardial infarction. The absence of Q waves along with other ECG findings can be of help in providing evidence for the presence of DCM. ECG findings can be varied or even normal but may include the presence of arrhythmias, such as, AF, sinus tachycardia, ventricular arrhythmias, AV conduction blocks and bundle branch blocks (complete or incomplete). The echocardiogram will provide proof of LV dilation/dysfunction. Not all causes for DCM are known, however viral infection (such as myocarditis), drugs and alcohol, pregnancy, neuromuscular disease (muscular dystrophies) and genetic familial factors are all potential causes.

## Hypertrophic Cardiomyopathy (HOCM/HCM)

Instead of dilation, the ventricular wall becomes thickened, or hypertrophied in the case of HOCM (Fig. 4.14). One of the first signs of this condition can be sudden cardiac death. Other symptoms can include angina, dyspnea and arrhythmias, including VT and VF. Atrial Fibrillation is also commonly seen in HOCM patients. Sometimes the thickened muscle can reduce the blood flow between the ventricle and aorta, termed an outflow tract obstruction. This can cause a turbulent blood flow, increasing the risk of clot formation.

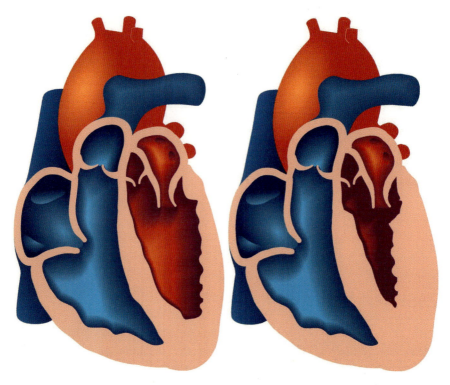

**Fig. 4.14**   Normal heart (*left*), LVH (*right*)

## *Takotsubo Cardiomyopathy*

Is a reversible left ventricular dysfunction that is triggered by sudden stress in a person with no previous history of coronary artery disease. The name takotsubo comes from Japan because the bulging apex of the heart resembled a takotsubo, a form of octopus trap (Fig. 4.15).

The condition often mimics symptoms of an acute coronary syndrome, including chest pain, raised troponin levels and ST segment elevation. Emotional stress, such as a recent death in the family or catastrophic medical diagnosis are believed to trigger the condition. One theory suggests that high levels of circulating catecholamines cause myocardial stunning and wall motion abnormalities. In turn the apex dilates and relaxes reducing cardiac contractility. In <20 % of cases the condition is triggered by physical causes, such as surgery, trauma and severe pain.

The condition is more common in females than males. Apical ballooning can be detected with LV angiography or contrast echocardiography. Treatment may include the use of a ventricular assist device, such as an IABP (Intra Aortic Balloon Pump). Placement of a temporary pacemaker is sometimes also used.

**Fig. 4.15** A Takotsubo

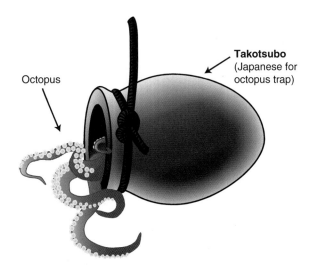

Octopus

**Takotsubo**
(Japanese for
octopus trap)

**Table 4.10** Interchangeable descriptions for Takotsubo cardiomyopathy

| Takotsubo alternative terms |
| --- |
| Broken heart syndrome |
| Stress induced cardiomyopathy |
| Transient apical ballooning syndrome |
| Ampulla cardiomyopathy |
| Stress cardiomyopathy |
| Gebrochenes-Herz-Syndrome |

ECG findings can often be confused with those found in a STEMI. There may be ST-segment elevation and/or other T wave inversion. A prolonged QT interval is sometimes present. As these findings are not sufficient to tell the difference between MI and Takotsubo cardiomyopathy, further tests, such as cardiac catheterization are required. A good patient history is also very helpful and may provide some initial clues. Takotsubo cardiomyopathy is also known by many other names as summarised in Table 4.10.

## *Arrhythmogenic Right Ventricular Dysplasia/ Cardiomyopathy (ARVD/C)*

ARVD/C is an inherited condition characterized by the presence of ventricular arrhythmia and right ventricular structural abnormalities. ARVD/C is also a leading cause of sudden cardiac death. One of the primary diagnostic criteria used to identify ARVD/C on the ECG is the presence of epsilon waves (Fig. 4.16.) which occur in around half of cases. Epsilon waves are waves that occur immediately after the

**Fig. 4.16** An epsilon wave
seen in lead II

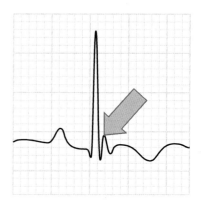

| Table 4.11 The signal average ECG | What is a signal averaged ECG? |
| --- | --- |
| | Signals are averaged to remove interference revealing what are termed as late ventricular potentials. These potentials allow practitioners to see minute QRS variations that may otherwise be obscured by interference on the surface ECG. |

QRS complex and are best seen in lead $V_1$, although they can often be difficult to see on surface ECGs. Signal averaged ECGs (Table 4.11) can be useful in the detection of epsilon waves. The other major finding is that of T wave inversion in the right precordial leads. Complete or incomplete RBBB is also often seen. In addition QRS prolongation in $V_1$–$V_3$ > 110 ms is seen, compared with the QRS duration in lead $V_6$. The condition can sometimes mimic Brugada syndrome (discussed in Chap. 8).

VT and VF are commonly seen in ARVD/C, as is a form of monomorphic VT called right ventricular outflow tract tachycardia (RVOT). RVOT is discussed in more detail in Chap. 6.

## Heart Failure

Heart failure, also known as congestive heart failure (CHF) is a condition where the heart muscle can no longer pump efficiently enough to perfuse the body efficiently. The condition often begins with one side of the heart. If one side of the heart starts to fail, failure of the other side is inevitable. In the initial stages of heart failure, symptoms can appear one-sided. Table 4.12 shows the common symptoms found in left and right sided heart failure. When both sides are affected, both sets of symptoms are present. As the condition progresses, the levels of functional disability and severity can be as great as those found in terminal lung cancer. Depression is also prevalent in heart failure cases and should not be overlooked by practitioners. Heart failure can be caused by many factors as summarised in Table 4.13. There is a blood test that can be used for the diagnosis of heart failure called a brain natriuretic peptide (BNP) or B-type natriuretic peptide. Levels of BNP >500 pg/ml are generally considered to be a positive indicator for heart failure (see Tables 4.14 and 4.15).

**Table 4.12** Some signs and symptoms of heart failure

| Right sided heart failure | Left sided heart failure |
| --- | --- |
| Shortness of breath | Shortness of breath |
| Peripheral oedema | Peripheral oedema |
| ↑ JVP (jugular venous pressure) | ↑ JVP (jugular venous pressure) |
| Palpitations | Tachypnea |
| Fatigue/weakness | Orthopnea |
| Ascites | Fatigue/weakness |
| Hepatomegaly (enlarged liver) | Cyanosis |
| Eczema-type rash on legs | Wheezing |
| Venous leg ulcers | Persistent cough |
| | ↓ urine output |
| | Weight gain (due to fluid retention) |
| | Weight loss in advanced cases |

**Table 4.13** Some of the causes of heart failure

| Causes of heart failure |
| --- |
| MI |
| Hypertension |
| Cardiomyopathy |
| Alcohol/drugs |
| Uncontrolled arrhythmia |
| Congenital cardiac conditions |
| Viral infection |
| Valve disease |

**Table 4.14** Physical examination in HF patients

| Full patient history |
| --- |
| Blood pressure |
| Pulse (rate, rhythm, quality) |
| Visual assessment (skin condition, oedema) |
| JVP |
| Assessment of apical pulse |
| Auscultation (listen to heart and lung sounds) |

Table 4.16 shows a functional classification of heart failure that is frequently used in clinical practice.

## Cardiac Resynchronization Therapy (CRT)

CRT also referred to as Biventricular pacing is one of the treatment options used to treat patients suffering from heart failure when they fulfil criteria for this treatment, as summarised in Table 4.17. CRT improves the pumping action of cardiac chambers by synchronizing their action improving cardiac output and LV ejection fraction. CRT works by introducing electrodes into the right atrium, right ventricle and

**Table 4.15** BNP levels (pg/ml)

| Brain natriuretic peptide/B-type natriuretic peptide | |
| --- | --- |
| < 100 | Normal |
| < 500 | Hospital discharge goal |
| ≥ 700 | Decompensated heart failure |

**Table 4.16** The New York Heart Association (NYHA) functional classification of heart failure

| Class | Effect | Description | Severity |
| --- | --- | --- | --- |
| I | No limitation | Ordinary physical activity but some evidence of heart failure, such as previous episodes or on treatment for heart failure. | N/A |
| II | Slight limitation | Comfortable at rest but shows symptoms with ordinary physical activity, such as: palpitations, fatigue dyspnoea or angina. | Mild |
| III | Marked limitation | Even low levels of activity cause symptoms but patient is still comfortable at rest. | Moderate |
| IV | Symptoms present at rest | Symptoms present even at rest, patient unable to perform any physical activity with discomfort. | Severe |

**Table 4.17** National Institute for Health and Clinical Excellence criteria for CRT

| NICE criteria for CRT |
| --- |
| NYHA symptom class III to IV |
| Patients in sinus rhythm with a QRS on ECG ≥150 ms or QRS of 120–149 ms with mechanical dyssynchrony confirmed by echocardiography |
| Left ventricular ejection fraction (LVEF) ≤35 % |
| Currently receiving optimal pharmacological therapy |

behind the left ventricle by means of the coronary sinus (Fig. 4.17). Leads are not placed directly into the left ventricle as there is a risk of thromboembolism and possible aortic valve impairment.

It is very difficult to distinguish between a biventricular pacemaker and a dual chamber pacemaker when looking at the ECG of a patient with a either pacemaker system. This is because both ventricles are synchronized, so there is only usually one spike visible before the QRS complex on the ECG. When looking at the ECG the practitioner could not be sure if they were looking at a dual chamber pacemaker or a biventricular pacemaker system (Fig. 4.18). Pacing and pacemakers are discussed in more detail in Chap. 5.

## Summary of Key Points

- There are several different evaluation methods for determining the presence of RVH and LVH varying in complexity. Practitioners should become familiar with a method(s) that they find easy to use/remember and are appropriate for their clinical setting

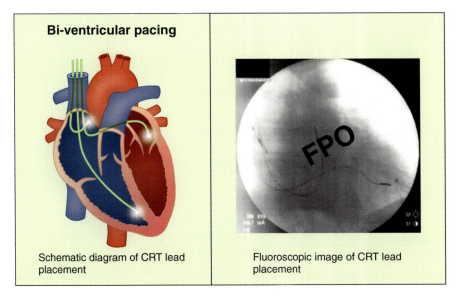

**Fig. 4.17** Schematic image of CRT lead placement (*left*), Fluoroscopic image of lead placement during insertion of a biventricular pacemaker for treatment of heart failure (*right*)

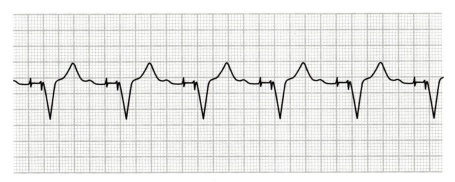

**Fig. 4.18** A dual chamber pacemaker (pacing spikes seen before both P wave and QRS complex)

- The term atrial abnormality is more accurate than atrial enlargement as we do not know the cause of the morphological changes
- Practitioners should state that voltage criteria has been met for a ventricular hypertrophy as other tests are required to confirm the diagnosis
- Cardiac resynchronization therapy/biventricular pacing is a treatment option for heart failure, provided patients meet certain criteria. It can be impossible to distinguish between dual chamber pacemaker systems and biventricular pacing systems on the ECG

# Quiz

Q1. Right atrial abnormality can be identified on the ECG by...
   (A) Pall peaked P waves >2.5 mm in amplitude
   (B) Wide bifid P waves >2.5 mm in width
   (C) Wide QRS complex >110 ms

Q2. Takotsubo cardiomyopathy often mimics ACS symptoms
   (A) True
   (B) False

Q3. Hypertrophy can be defined as...
   (A) Tall R waves
   (B) An increase in the amount of cells in an organ or tissue.
   (C) An increase in the size of cells leading to the enlargement of an organ or
       tissue.

Q4. Epsilon waves are sometimes seen in...
   (A) Hypertrophic cardiomyopathy
   (B) Takotsubo cardiomyopathy
   (C) Arrhythmogenic Right Ventricular Dysplasia/Cardiomyopathy (ARVD/C)

Q5. The difference between a dual chamber pacemaker system and a biventricular
   system is identified on the ECG...
   (A) By narrow R waves
   (B) It is often impossible to tell the difference
   (C) Bifid P waves

Identify the following ECGs

**Q6.**

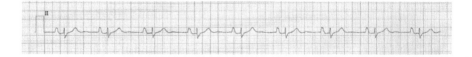

**Q7.**

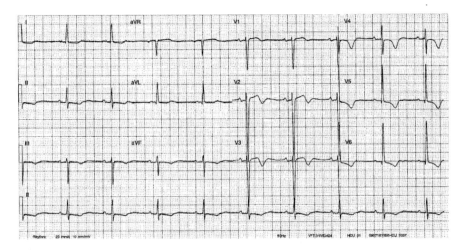

**Q8.**

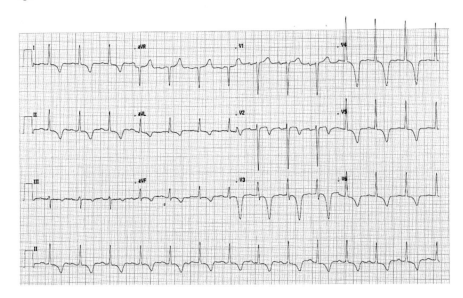

**Q9.**

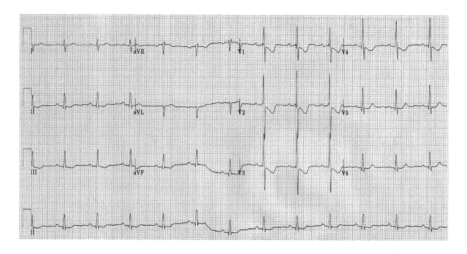

Answers: Q1 = A, Q2 = A, Q3 = C, Q4 = C, Q5 = B, Q6 = Right atrial abnormality, Q7 = LVH + 'strain pattern', Q8 = LVH + 'strain pattern', Q9 = RVH

# Chapter 5
# Conduction Blocks and Cardiac Pacing

**Keywords** Heart block • AV block • SA block • Pacemakers • Pacing • Bundle branch blocks

## Background

Any part of the conduction system can be blocked preventing or delaying impulses reaching subsequent parts of the conduction system. These blocks should be classified as conduction delays or blocks, not as arrhythmias even though they can cause the appearance of rhythm irregularities.

## Bundle Branch Blocks

A bundle branch block refers to the blocking of the electrical impulse down one of the bundle branches (Fig. 5.1), referred to as a left bundle branch block (LBBB) or a right bundle branch block (RBBB).

Disease or damage of the conduction system can result in a bundle branch block. Table 5.1 shows some of the common causes for bundle branch blocks.

The salient feature seen in both left and right bundle branch blocks are the presence of widened QRS complexes in all leads (a QRS duration of >0.10 s/2.5 small squares). With this in mind it is also necessary to consider and rule out other causes of QRS prolongation, including; ventricular paced rhythms, idioventricular rhythm, broad complex tachycardia and premature ventricular beats.

### Right Bundle Branch Blocks

A RBBB (Fig. 5.2) is often seen in older patients and does not require treatment. The best leads to use for the identification of a RBBB are $V_1$ and $V_6$. The QRS duration needs to exceed 120 ms/0.12 s. Normal septal depolarization occurs, followed by depolarization of the left bundle branch and then the right; due to the block the

© Springer-Verlag London 2015
A. Davies, A. Scott, *Starting to Read ECGs: A Comprehensive Guide to Theory and Practice*, DOI 10.1007/978-1-4471-4965-1_5

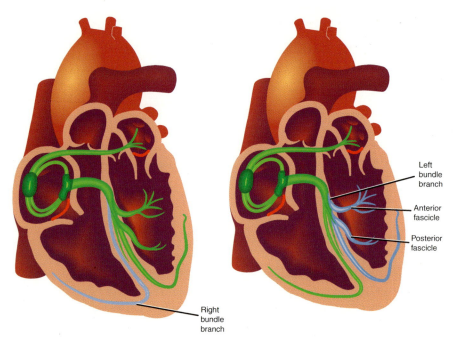

**Fig. 5.1**  The right and left bundle branches

**Table 5.1**  Causes of bundle branch blocks

| |
| --- |
| Ischemic heart disease |
| Myocardial infarction |
| Cardiomyopathy |
| Fibrosis of the conduction system |
| Hypertension |
| Pulmonary embolism |
| Atrial septal defect |
| Other congenital heart disease |
| Normal variant |

impulse then travels through the slower myocardial tissue, leading to an increase in QRS duration. Repolarization is affected by the abnormal depolarization, so the T wave is deflected in the opposite direction to the terminal portion of the QRS complex. Table 5.2 shows the changes seen in leads $V_1$ and $V_6$ forming the rsR pattern in $V_1$ and qRS pattern in $V_6$.

**Incomplete Right Bundle Branch Block**

When the morphological changes for a RBBB exist and the QRS duration is >100 ms but <120 ms, it is referred to as an incomplete right bundle branch block.

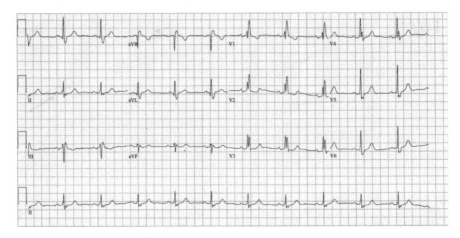

**Fig. 5.2** A right bundle branch block

| **Table 5.2** Changes seen in leads $V_1$ and $V_6$ in the presence of a RBBB | $V_1$ | $V_6$ |
|---|---|---|
| | Small r wave | Small q wave |
| | s wave | Tall R wave |
| | Secondary R wave | Deep S wave |
| | T wave deflected in opposite direction of the terminal portion of the QRS complex | T wave deflected in opposite direction of the terminal portion of the QRS complex |

## *Left Bundle Branch Blocks*

Left bundle branch blocks (Fig. 5.3) are not often seen in healthy individuals and are often associated with chronic coronary heart disease. In a LBBB the septal depolarization takes place from the right to the left. Left ventricular depolarisation is carried out through the slower myocardial tissue increasing the QRS duration. As with a RBBB leads $V_1$ and $V_6$ are the best leads to view for changes associated with a LBBB (Table 5.3).

Patients with advanced disease of the conduction system and coronary heart disease often present with a LBBB and an axis deviation. These changes are associated with increased mortality.

If a patient presents with chest pain and new LBBB they should be treated as a medical emergency and undergo cardiac catheterisation or thrombolysis according to local policy. As a LBBB has associated ST elevation and Q waves, the ECG becomes a less reliable indicator of myocardial infarction.

Sgarbossa's criteria is a point based system to help identify the possibility of a STEMI in patients with a LBBB (Table 5.4). A score of three or more suggests the presence of a STEMI. The use of serial ECGs and the examination of primary T wave changes are generally more sensitive than the criteria.

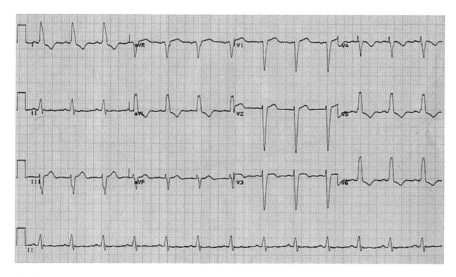

**Fig. 5.3**  A left bundle branch block

**Table 5.3**  Changes seen in leads $V_1$ and $V_6$ in the presence of a LBBB

| $V_1$ | $V_6$ |
|---|---|
| QS or rS pattern | No q waves |
| Small r wave in around 30 % of cases | Notched R wave |
| Positive notch present following Q wave | Negative notch following R wave |
| T wave deflected in opposite direction to the QRS complex | T wave deflected in opposite direction to the QRS complex |

**Table 5.4**  Sgarbossa's criteria for detecting acute myocardial infarction in the presence of LBBB

| Criteria | Points |
|---|---|
| ST elevation ≥1 mm in a lead with positively deflected QRS complexes | 5 |
| ST elevation ≥5 mm in a lead with negatively deflected QRS complexes | 2 |
| ST depression ≥1 mm in lead $V_1/V_2/V_3$ | 3 |

**Incomplete Left Bundle Branch Block**

An incomplete left bundle branch block has the same morphology as a LBBB with the exception of the QRS duration, which is less than 120 ms/0.12 s.

## Rate Dependent/Transient Bundle Branch Blocks

It is also possible for a bundle branch block to appear intermittently. Infection, cardiac catheterization, MI and heart failure are known causative factors. There is also a form of rate dependant bundle branch block that is caused when a rapid heart rate does not allow the bundle branch time to recover and is still in a refractory state, preventing the next impulse passing through the bundle branch.

## *Features and Criteria for Identifying Left and Right Bundle Branch Blocks*

There are several features that help practitioners tell the difference between a left and right bundle branch block as summarised in Table 5.5.

## *William Morrow/William Marrow*

Is a mnemonic often taught to help practitioners remember the key features of left and right bundle branch blocks. Essentially the first and last letter show the deflection of the QRS complex in leads $V_1$ and $V_6$ respectively with 'W' being negatively deflected and 'M' being positively defected. The 'LL' in WilLLam=LBBB, the 'RR' in MaRRow or MoRRow=RBBB. Table 5.6 shows an example of this.

## *Hemiblocks*

If a patient presents with a RBBB and left or right axis deviation, one of the fascicles of the left bundle branch is also blocked. A block in the anterior or posterior fascicles of the left bundle branch is termed a hemiblock. The direction of axis deviation tells the practitioner if the block is in the left anterior or posterior fascicle, as demonstrated in Table 5.7. When a RBBB exists with a hemiblock, it is termed a

**Table 5.5** Features of left and right bundle branch blocks

| LBBB | RBBB |
|---|---|
| QRS negatively deflected in $V_1$ | QRS positively deflected in $V_1$ |
| Widened QRS complexes in all leads | Widened QRS complexes in all leads |
| QS pattern in $V_1$ | rsR pattern in $V_1$ |
| T-wave inversion in $V_6$ | qRS pattern in $V_6$ |
| ST-segment elevation (sometimes) seen in $V_1$–$V_4$ | T-wave inversion in $V_6$ |

**Table 5.6** The mnemonic William Marrow/Morrow

|  | QRS deflection in $V_1$ |  | Left/right block |  |  | QRS deflection in $V_6$ |
|---|---|---|---|---|---|---|
| **LBBB** | W | i | LL | i | a | M |
| **RBBB** | M | o/a | RR | o |  | W |

**Table 5.7** Left anterior and posterior hemiblocks (with additional features)

| Left anterior hemiblock | Left posterior hemiblock |
|---|---|
| RBBB + left axis | RBBB + right axis |
| Left axis deviation ≥ −40° | Right axis deviation ≥ 120° |
| qR pattern in lead I | rS pattern in lead I |
| rS pattern in lead II | qR pattern in lead II (without right ventricular hypertrophy criteria) |

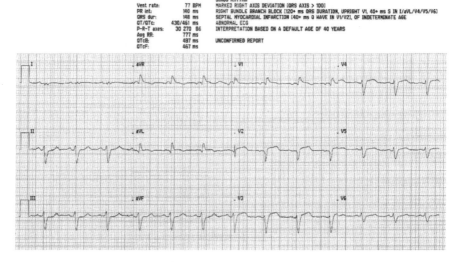

**Fig. 5.4** Example of a bifascicular block (RBBB + right axis deviation = left posterior hemiblock)

bifascicular block (Fig. 5.4). A LBBB is a form of bifascicular block as both fascicles of the left bundle are blocked.

## Trifascicular Block

Trifascicular block refers to a blockage of all three fascicles and is a bilateral bundle branch block. There are two types of trifascicular block, complete or incomplete. A complete trifascicular block is caused by a RBBB that leads to 3rd degree AV nodal block or ventricular standstill. AV nodal blocks are discussed later in the chapter in the section about AV blocks. An incomplete trifascicular block (Fig. 5.5) however is detected by the presence of a bifascicular block with a 1st degree AV nodal block (also discussed later in the chapter).

## Atrioventricular Nodal Blocks

AV nodal blocks are blocks that inhibit the ability of the AV node to conduct an impulse to the subsequent conduction system. There are three main types of AV block,

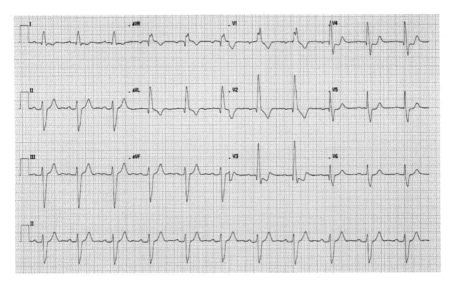

**Fig. 5.5** An incomplete trifascicular block (RBBB + right axis deviation + 1st degree AV block)

known as; 1st, 2nd and 3rd degree AV nodal block. These blocks can either be permanent or temporary. AV blocks are best seen by examining the ECGs rhythm strip.

## 1st Degree AV Block

This form of block does not normally require treatment, it is identified by a delay between atrial depolarization and ventricular depolarisation, seen on the ECG as an increase in the PR interval >200 ms/0.20s (5 small squares) (Fig. 5.6). Although the PR interval is increased, the increase is the same for each beat (Fig. 5.7). Each P wave is followed by a QRS complex and the rhythm is usually regular. Causes of 1st degree AV block are summarized in Table 5.8.

## 2nd Degree AV Block

Second degree AV block is further divided into two subtypes, known as type I and type II 2nd degree AV block.

### 2nd Degree AV Block (Type I)

2nd degree AV block type I, also known as Mobitz type I can be identified on the ECG by a PR interval that increases duration with every subsequent beat until a P wave is seen without a subsequent QRS complex (a dropped beat). The cycle then

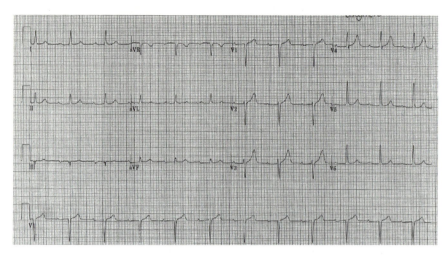

**Fig. 5.6**  A 12-lead ECG showing 1st degree AV block (prolonged PR interval best seen in rhythm srip, lead V₁)

**Fig. 5.7**  Long PR interval
(the same length in each beat)

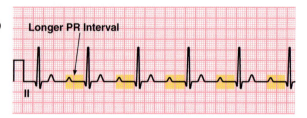

| **Table 5.8**  Common causes of 1st degree AV block | |
| --- | --- |
| | Normal variant |
| | Ischemic heart disease |
| | Increased vagal tone |
| | Drugs that prolong AV conduction time (i.e. Beta Blockers) |
| | Fibrosis of the conduction system |
| | Acute MI |

repeats. This leads to the appearance of grouped QRS complexes on the rhythm strip of the ECG. There is often a pattern to the irregularity of the rhythm. The number of P waves to QRS complexes can be expressed as a ratio of P to QRS or can be variable. The progressive lengthening of the PR interval is referred to as Wenckebach phenomenon (Figs. 5.8 and 5.9).

Sometimes 2nd degree AV block type I is referred to as 'Wenckebach block'. This is a potentially misleading description. Wenckebach phenomenon is the dropping of a beat following a progressive lengthening of conduction time in any cardiac tissue. As such this phenomenon doesn't just apply to the AV node.

**Fig. 5.8** Increasing PR interval (Wenckebach phenomenon)

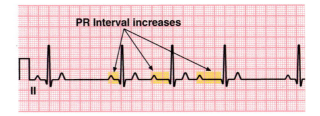

**PR Interval increases**

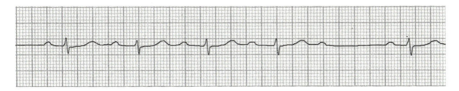

**Fig. 5.9** 2nd degree AV block (type I) [Life in the Fast Lane (http://lifeinthefastlane.com/education/procedures/lead-positioning/)/CC BY-SA 4.0 (http://creativecommons.org/licenses/by-sa/4.0/)]

**Table 5.9** Common causes of 2nd degree AV block (type I)

| |
| --- |
| Normal variant |
| Ischemic heart disease |
| Drugs that prolong AV conduction time (i.e. Beta Blockers) |
| Atrial septal defect |
| Acute MI |
| Mitral valve prolapse |
| Aortic valve disease |

The progressively lengthening PR interval is caused by successive impulses arriving in the AV node whilst it is in its relative refractory period. The earlier the impulse arrives during the refractory period, the longer it will take to pass through the node to the subsequent conduction system. If the impulse arrives during the absolute refractory period, the impulse will not be transmitted to the ventricles, this leads to the appearance of a P wave with no subsequent QRS complex on the ECG. Common causes of 2nd degree AV block are listed in Table 5.9. A significant number of people experience this block transiently during sleep. If the block is present when the patient is awake and is symptomatic, consideration should be given to pacemaker insertion.

## 2nd Degree AV Block (Type II)

This subtype of 2nd degree AV block, also known as Mobitz type II carries a worse prognosis and can lead to complete heart block. The block occurs lower down in the bundle branches or the bundle of His and is a form of intermittent bilateral bundle

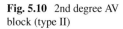

**Fig. 5.10**  2nd degree AV
block (type II)

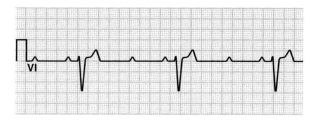

**Table 5.10**  Common causes
of 2nd degree AV block
(type II)

| |
| --- |
| Normal variant |
| Cardiomyopathy |
| Coronary artery disease |
| Fibrosis of the conduction system |
| MI (usually anterior wall) |

branch block. In this instance the PR interval is the same length but occasionally there will be a P wave with no subsequent QRS complex. This is caused by the intermittent bilateral bundle branch block preventing the impulse activating the ventricles after the atria, hence the P wave with no following QRS (Fig. 5.10). The block is often seen in the presence of an existing bundle branch block and may occur intermittently causing an irregular rhythm, or it may occur consistently, causing a regular rhythm. It can be difficult to differentiate between type I and type II block if there are less than two consecutively conducted P waves present. Several nonconducted P waves in succession termed high grade block are usually an indication for cardiac pacing. Common causes of 2nd degree AV block (type II) are listed in Table 5.10.

## *3rd Degree AV Block*

Otherwise known as complete heart block. This indicates that no atrial impulses are conducted to the ventricles. To prevent the heart going into ventricular standstill an impulse can be generated further down the conduction system as a safety net. This is referred to as an escape beat. Narrow QRS complexes <50 bpm are junctional escape beats, slower wider QRS complexes (<40 bpm) are ventricular escape beats. The P waves and QRS complexes are usually regular but have no relationship with each other (complete A/V dissociation). Figure 5.11 shows this dyssynchrony in action. There are regular P waves (the first few highlighted by arrows), there are also regular escape beats. There is no relationship between the two. P waves are seen before, after and during the QRS complexes, failing to trigger the ventricles. The regular escape beat prevents ventricular standstill, but is much slower than a regular heartbeat at approximately 40 BPM in this case. Patients with this block may present with hypotension and collapse (sometimes called Stokes-Adams attacks). Pacing is often used as a treatment for patients presenting with complete heart block. Common causes of complete heart block are listed in Table 5.11.

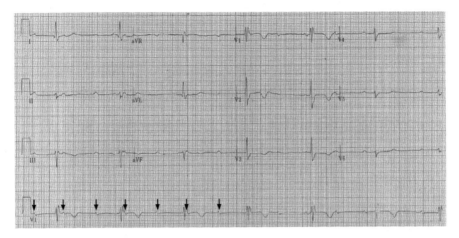

**Fig. 5.11** 3rd degree AV block

**Table 5.11** Common causes of 3rd degree AV block

| |
|---|
| Normal variant |
| Ischemic heart disease |
| Increased vagal tone |
| Drugs that prolong AV conduction time (i.e. Beta Blockers) |
| Congenital heart disease |
| Fibrosis of the conduction system |
| Acute MI |

## *3rd Degree AV Block and Atrial Fibrillation*

Atrial fibrillation (AF) is usually defined as an irregularly irregular rhythm with no visible P waves. There is an exception to this when 3rd degree AV block and AF are present at the same time. Figure 5.12 shows an example of this. No P waves are visible and the characteristic chaotic undulating baseline of AF can be seen. The ventricular rhythm however is regular. This is because none of the impulses generated by the ectopic foci causing the AF are transmitted to the ventricles and the resulting escape beat generated further down the conduction system is unaffected and thus regular.

A medication review should also be carried out when presented with a patient with an AV block as drugs that prolong AV conduction time, such as Beta Blockers can cause AV block. 2nd and 3rd degree AV blocks should only be considered in the presence of an appropriate atrial rate. Rates above 250 beats per minute cause the AV node to prevent conduction and drop beats as a protective mechanism to prevent the ventricular rate continuing to rise making the patient hemodynamically unstable.

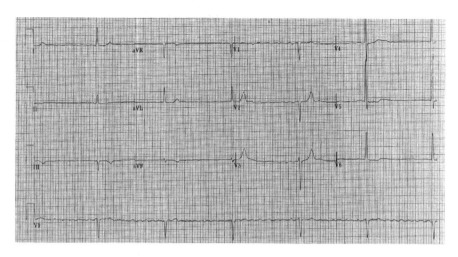

**Fig. 5.12**  3rd degree AV block and AF

## Sinoatrial Block

Is identified on the ECG by the lack of P waves. SA block can be complete or incomplete. Incomplete SA block causes the occasional loss of P waves, whereas complete SA block prevents any impulses leaving the SA node, causing sinus arrest (a lack of any heart beats). These blocks are subdivided in the same was as AV nodal blocks.

## *1st Degree SA Block*

1st degree SA block is caused by an action potential delay between the SA node and the atria. As such this block is impossible to see on the surface ECG because the ECG does not show the firing of the SA node. 1st degree SA block can however be detected during electrophysiology studies.

## *2nd Degree SA Block*

### 2nd Degree SA Block (Type I)

Seen on the ECG as a gradual reduction in the P to P interval resulting in an eventual pause and then a repeat of the cycle. Figure 5.13 shows this in action, a progressively shortening P to P interval resulting in no subsequent PQRST wave (a pause) on the ECG.

**Fig. 5.13** 2nd degree SA block, type I (also known as type I sinus exit block)

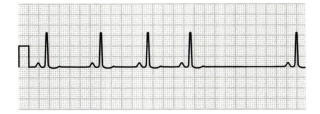

**Fig. 5.14** 2nd degree SA block, type II (also known as type II sinus exit block)

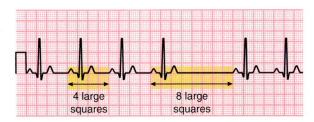

4 large squares     8 large squares

## 2nd Degree SA Block (Type II)

Is determined due to its mathematical relationship with the conduction cycle. In this type of SA block there is no shortening of the P to P interval, instead there is an unexpected absence of a P wave and subsequent QRS complex. The pause is multiple of the P to P interval. Figure 5.14 shows an example of this using large squares as the measure to make them easier to see. Measuring from the start of one P wave to the start of the next (the P to P interval) before the pause is 4 large squares, measuring the P to P interval of the beats before and after the pause is 8 large squares. Eight is a multiple of 4.

## *3rd Degree SA Block*

Also known as complete SA block or sinus arrest has no mathematical relationship with pauses lasting up to several seconds. Patients can become hemodynamically unstable and collapse depending on the length of the pause. As with 3rd degree AV block, escape beats are usually triggered to prevent asystole. The morphology of the escape beat can give clues to its origin (junctional or ventricular). As shown in Fig. 5.15, which depicts a long pause followed by a junctional escape beat.

There are four main causes for the absence of P waves on an ECG, including:

- Failure of the impulse to leave the sinoatrial node.
- Failure of the sinoatrial node to generate an impulse
- Impulse is inadequate and fails to activate the atria
- Atrial paralysis (prevents atrial activation)

**Fig. 5.15** 3rd degree SA block (also known as complete SA block)

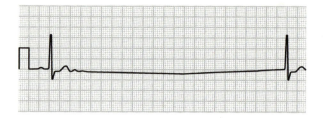

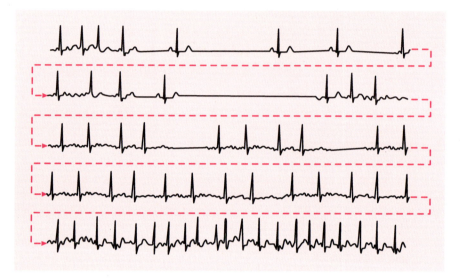

**Fig. 5.16** Sick sinus syndrome (taken from a continuous rhythm strip)

## Sick Sinus Syndrome

The term 'sick sinus syndrome' describes a situation where marked sinus bradycardia and periods of sinoatrial block/arrest coexist with periods of tachycardia, called brady-tachy syndrome (Fig. 5.16).

The problem with the term 'sick sinus syndrome' is that it implies that the sole source of the problem lies with the sinus node. If this was the case, then any prolonged pause of a few seconds would be prevented earlier by escape beats, generated from further down the conduction system. The problem affects more of the conduction system than just the sinus node. Prolonged atrial pauses are likely to be caused by impairment of impulse forming cells and/or enhanced parasympathetic activity. Atrial fibrillation/flutter can also be seen on the ECG, triggering the tachycardia. Most patients presenting with sick sinus syndrome may have normal sinus rhythm with intermittent bouts of sinus bradycardia, SA block/arrest, escape beats or rhythms and brady-tachy syndrome. Table 5.12 shows the common causes of sick sinus syndrome.

**Table 5.12** Common causes of sick sinus syndrome

| |
| --- |
| Fibrosis of the SAN |
| Cardiomyopathy |
| Ischemic heart disease |
| Drugs (i.e. digoxin, Beta Blockers, calcium channel blockers) |
| Damage to the SAN caused by surgery |
| Inflammatory cardiac disease |

**Table 5.13** Summary of temporary pacing methods

| Pacing method | Description |
| --- | --- |
| Transvenous | The most commonly used form of temporary pacing. A lead is passed into the right atrium or ventricle via a vein, often the subclavian or internal jugular. |
| Epicardial | Used during cardiac surgery, leads are placed directly onto the epicardium during open heart surgery. |
| Transcutaneous/ transthoracic | This is a non-invasive method of pacing in an emergency. Using a defibrillator as a pulse generator, ECG electrodes are applied to the patient along with the standard defibrillator pads. The practitioner then chooses how much electricity in mA (milliamps) to use to pace the heart effectively. The practitioner looks for a pacing spike followed by a wide QRS complex to determine that have achieved capture. The patients pulse should also be checked manually to confirm the effectiveness. |

# Cardiac Pacing

Patients experiencing reduced cardiac output as a result of a conduction block or other damage to the conduction system may require cardiac pacing. Pacemakers work by emitting an electrical pulse from a pulse generator (essentially a battery) to the myocardium via a pacing lead(s). The impulse triggers activation of one or more of the heart's chambers as required. There are several different types of pacemaker that are used in different situations. These can be broadly split into two main types: temporary (Table 5.13) and permanent pacemakers. Temporary pacing is often used in emergencies or to treat a condition until a permanent pacemaker system can be implanted. Temporary pacemakers are often inserted at the patients bedside, permanent systems are usually inserted in a pacing/catheterization lab or operating theatre.

There are also several types of permanent pacemaker system described by which chambers they pace, they are:

- Single chamber pacing (atrium or ventricle)
- Dual chamber/sequential A-V pacing
- Biventricular pacing/CRT

Permanent pacemaker leads are often introduced via the cephalic or subclavian veins using fluoroscopic imaging (Fig. 5.17). The pulse generator is located

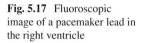
**Fig. 5.17** Fluoroscopic image of a pacemaker lead in the right ventricle

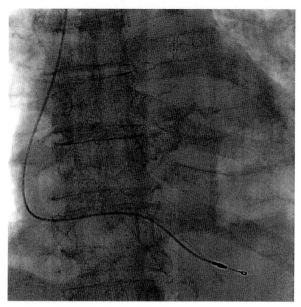

in a pacemaker pocket made by creating a small incision in the pectoralis fascia around an inch below the clavicle (Fig. 5.18). Most pacemaker pockets are located on the non-dominant side (i.e. if the patient is right handed the pocket will located on the left side of the body). Sometimes different pocket positions can be used. An example of this is the retromammary technique (Fig. 5.19) that is used often with young women who may be more concerned about the scar left after pocket closure. This technique helps to hide the scar and the device so they are not visible.

## Understanding Pacing Codes

Pacing codes are often used to describe the functions of permanent pacemakers. A summary of the commonly encountered codes are seen in Table 5.14.

For example two commonly encountered pacemaker codes, VVI and DDDR offer a lot of information about the type of pacemaker system the patient has. VVI tells us that the ventricle is paced, the second letter tells us that the ventricle is the chamber that is used to sense the impulse. The 'I' refers to the response used based on the result of sensing. In this case inhibited. This means that if the pacemaker detects the patients natural heartbeat it doesn't need to do anything, i.e. it inhibits (prevents) the pacemaker responding by generating an impulse, as it is not

**Fig. 5.18** Permanent
pacemaker pocket (standard
location)

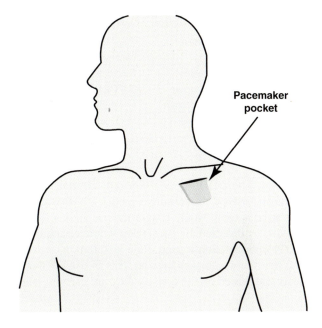

Pacemaker
pocket

**Fig. 5.19** The retromammary
technique

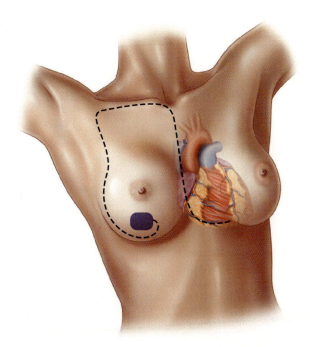

**Table 5.14** Commonly used pacemaker codes

| Chamber(s) paced | Chamber(s) sensed | Sensing response | Rate modulation | Multisite pacing |
|---|---|---|---|---|
| 0=None | 0=None | 0=None | 0=None | 0=None |
| A=Atrium | A=Atrium | T=Triggered | R=Rate modulation | A=Atrium |
| V=Ventricle | V=Ventricle | I=Inhibited | | V=Ventricle |
| D=Dual (A+V) | D=Dual (A+V) | D=Dual (T+I) | | D=Dual (A+V) |

required. The DDDR pacemaker tells us that both the atrium and ventricle are paced and sensed, the sensing response is both triggered and inhibited. This means that atrial activity would trigger the pacemaker, however if atrial and ventricular activity are detected the pacemaker would be inhibited. The final letter 'R' means that rate modulation is used. Rate modulation essentially changes the target heart rate that the pacemaker fires at. This is used if the patient requires a change in heart rate, based on the activity they are carrying out, such as exercise, climbing stairs etc.

## *Single Chamber Pacemakers*

As the name implies, a single chamber pacemaker only paces a single chamber of the heart. This can be either the atrium or ventricle. One of the issues with single chamber ventricular pacemakers in the loss of 'atrial kick'. This type of pacemaker is often used for sedentary patients.

### Loss of Atrial Kick

Atrial kick is the effect of atrial contraction preceding ventricular systole that improves the ventricular ejection fraction. When a single chamber pacemaker is used to pace the ventricle, the extra contribution from the atrium known as 'atrial kick' may be lost. This can reduce cardiac output by (15–30 %). The lack of synchronization between the atria and ventricles can also lead to insufficiency of the mitral and tricuspid valves.

Figure 5.20 shows the loss of 'atrial kick' in action, the ECG rhythm is shown above with the patients intrinsic rhythm followed by several paced beats identified by their wide QRS complexes. Directly below the ECG the patients arterial pressure can be seen. The pressure waveform is dampened during ventricular pacing showing reduced pressure as a result of the loss of atrial kick.

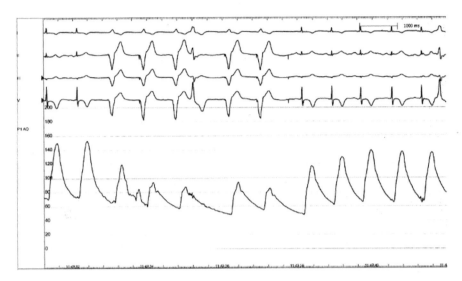

**Fig. 5.20** Intrinsic and paced rhythm showing the effect of loss of atrial kick on the pressure waveform

**Table 5.15** Two criteria for evaluating a maximum heart rate for signs of chronotropic incompetence

| Chronotropic incompetence |
| --- |
| Maximum heart rate during exercise <90 % of (220 – patients age) |
| OR |
| Maximum heart rate during exercise <120 bpm |

### Chronotropic Incompetence

This is a condition where the patients heart rate cannot increase fast enough to meet their metabolic requirements. This can manifest in several different ways, including: a delay or failure in achieving maximum heart rate and/or an inadequacy in maximum rate or recovering heart rate when exercising (Table 5.15).

## Dual Chamber Pacemakers

Dual chamber systems are often given to younger and/or more active patients, as they are shown to improve exercise capacity over single chamber chamber devices. Dual chamber systems often detect atrial activity and activate the ventricle if subsequent ventricular activity doesn't take place automatically. This helps to maintain A-V synchrony.

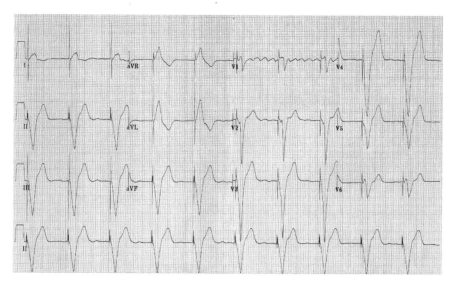

**Fig. 5.21**  ECG showing the characteristic pacing spikes followed by wide QRS complexes indicative of ventricular pacing

**Fig. 5.22**  Single chamber ventricular pacing (pacing spikes before QRS complexes)

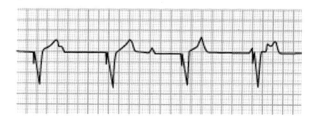

## Biventricular Pacemakers

Also known as cardiac resynchronization therapy (CRT) is used as a treatment for heart failure for patients who fulfil certain criteria. Biventricular pacemakers are discussed in more detail on Chap. 4.

## Pacemakers and the ECG

Pacing spikes, sometimes called pacing artifacts are the key feature seen on the 12-lead ECG with individuals who have a pacemaker system. Pacing spikes are vertical lines that precede QRS complexes (Fig. 5.21), P waves or both (Figs. 5.22 and 5.23). Sometimes pacing spikes can be subtle and more difficult to spot. These spikes are the result of the electrical impulse generated by the pacemaker that are visible on the ECG. They are narrow because the impulse has a very short duration (around 0.4 ms).

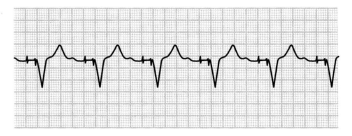

**Fig. 5.23** Dual chamber pacemaker (pacing spikes before both P waves and QRS complexes)

**Table 5.16** Poles found in an electrical circuit

| Positive pole (+) | Negative pole (−) |
| --- | --- |
| Anode | Cathode |

Electrical circuits are made of two poles (Table 5.16). Unipolar leads have a single pole on the pacing lead. Because this forms a large circuit, pacing spikes on the surface ECG are large. In contrast to this; bipolar leads have both poles on the lead, making a much smaller circuit with smaller packing spikes.

## *Pacemaker Problems Visible on the ECG*

The ECG can also be used to identify various problems with pacemaker systems (Table 5.17), including:

- Failure to sense
- Failure to capture
- Failure to pace
- Oversensing

## Summary of Key Points

- Impulse blocks can occur in any part of the conduction system. The location of the block can be determined with the ECG
- A new LBBB and chest pain should be treated as a medical emergency
- Pacing spikes/artefact are the salient feature of an artificial electronic pacemaker
- Pacemaker codes can be used to determine the type of pacemaker system the patient has
- Pacemakers are often used to treat conduction blocks
- Identification of some pacemaker problems are possible using the ECG

**Table 5.17** Commonly encountered pacemaker malfunctions

| Malfunction | Explanation | Surface ECG findings |
|---|---|---|
| Failure to sense | Pacemaker not sensing the patients intrinsic rhythm and firing. This is potentially dangerous as a pacing spike landing on a T wave can trigger 'R on T' phenomenon, leading to VT/VF. | Pacing spikes at various locations in the patients intrinsic cardiac cycle |
| Failure to capture | Firing of the pacemaker occurs but does not lead to subsequent chamber activation. The patient is then exposed to the condition that the pacemaker was inserted to treat. | Presence of pacing spikes with no subsequent waveform |
| Failure to pace | The pacemaker fails to pace when it should. This can lead to reduced cardiac output. | Gaps on the ECG between complexes where pacing activity would otherwise be expected |
| Oversensing | An oversensitivity of the pacemaker picks up muscular or other movement and mistakes it as part of the cardiac cycle and subsequently doesn't trigger impulse generation. | Insufficient or no pacemaker activity is seen on the ECG. |

# Quiz

- Q1. A regular prolonged PR interval of the same length for each beat is a sign of.
  - (A) Complete heart block
  - (B) 1st degree AV node block
  - (C) 2nd degree type I AV node block

- Q2. $V_1$ is positively deflected in a LBBB
  - (A) True
  - (B) False

- Q3. Loss of atrial kick
  - (A) Reduces cardiac output
  - (B) Increases cardiac output
  - (C) Increases the PR interval

- Q4. Paced ventricular rhythms on the ECG can be identified by.
  - (A) Pacing spikes before the P wave, followed by no QRS complex
  - (B) Pacing spikes before the QRS complex, followed by a wide QRS complex
  - (C) Pacing spikes before the QRS complex, followed by a narrow QRS complex

- Q5. The ventricular rhythm in ECGs with AF and complete heart block is
  - (A) Irregular
  - (B) Regular

- Q6. Patients with 2nd degree AV nodal block should be given an extra large dose of beta blockers
  - (A) True
  - (B) False

Interpret the following ECGs.

**Q7.**

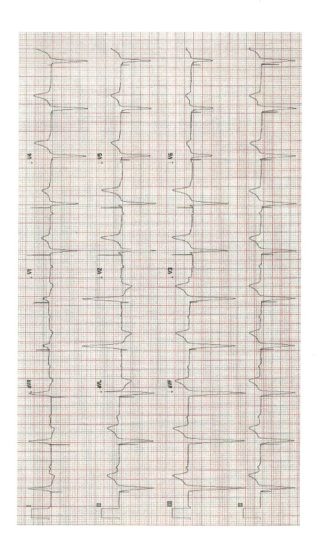

**Q8.**

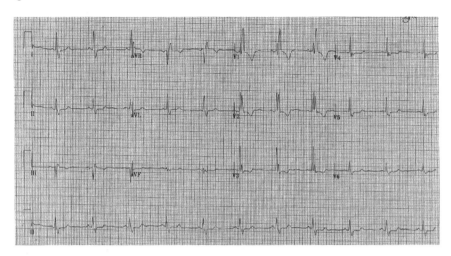

**Q9.**

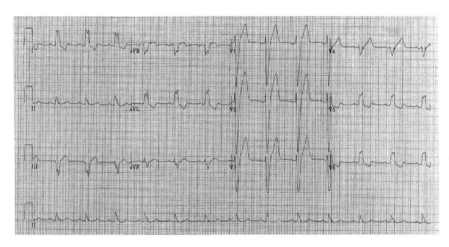

- Answers: Q1 = B, Q2 = B, Q3 = A, Q4 = B, Q5 = B, Q6 = B, Q7 = Ventricular paced rhythm, Q8 = RBBB, Q9 = LBBB

# Chapter 6
# Arrhythmias

**Keywords** Tachycardia • Fibrillation • Supraventricular • Rhythm • Arrhythmia • Ectopic • Premature beat • Polymorphic • Bigeminy • Trigeminy • Flutter • Reentry

## Background

The word arrhythmia derives from the Greek to mean loss or absence of rhythm. Essentially an arrhythmia is an irregular heartbeat and includes tachyarrhythmias and bradyarrhythmias. Abnormal electrical impulse conduction causes arrhythmias. There are several mechanisms of arrhythmia genesis, including; triggered activity, abnormal/enhanced automaticity, reentry and conduction delays. These mechanisms are discussed in more detail below with the exception of conduction delays, which are discussed in detail in Chap. 5. As many arrhythmias are caused by or sustained by ectopic foci it is necessary to gain an understanding of ectopy.

## Premature Beats

The term premature beat more accurately describes ectopic beats. Premature beats can originate from the atrial, junctional or ventricular regions of the heart. The most salient feature of a premature beat is a beat that occurs earlier than expected in the cardiac cycle and has a different morphology to the normal underlying rhythm (Fig. 6.1). The morphological changes are the key way of identifying the origin of a premature beat. The main differences between the different types of premature beat are summarised in Table 6.1.

© Springer-Verlag London 2015
A. Davies, A. Scott, *Starting to Read ECGs: A Comprehensive Guide to Theory and Practice*, DOI 10.1007/978-1-4471-4965-1_6

**Fig. 6.1**  A ventricular
premature beat

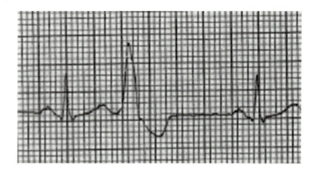

**Table 6.1**  The primary features of premature beats

| Atrial premature beat (APB) | Junctional premature beat (JPB) | Ventricular premature beat (VPB) |
|---|---|---|
| Normal beat    Atrial premature beat | Inverted p wave | |
| A beat occurring earlier than expected with a P wave morphology differing from patients normal P wave | A beat occurring earlier than expected with no visible P wave. Alternatively the P wave may appear inverted and may occur before or after the QRS complex. | A beat occurring earlier than expected with a wide bizarre QRS complex. The T wave is usually in the opposite direction to the terminal portion of the QRS complex. |

## *Premature Beat Origin*

There are three primary mechanisms that are considered to be the cause of premature beats, they consist of:

- Enhanced automaticity
  - Changes in the cellular threshold level increasing diastolic depolarization
    leading to premature beat formation
- Triggered activity
  - Damage to the myocardium can result in oscillation of the transmembrane
    potential. Leakage of positive ions into the cell creates after depolarizations
    leading to premature beats. Arrhythmias seen in Digoxin toxicity and long QT
    syndromes are thought to be caused by triggered activity
- Reentry circuits/circus movement
  - Discussed in more detail later in the chapter

## Compensatory and Non-compensatory Pauses

Compensatory pauses are temporary interruptions of sinus rhythm by a 'gap' or 'pause' with a duration that is a multiple of the normal cardiac cycle. To measure a compensatory pause, take three consecutive PQRST complexes from an otherwise regular rhythm. Measure the distance between the start of the first P wave of the first beat to the start of the P wave of the third beat. Next measure the same distance starting with the start of the P wave from the normal beat before the premature beat and ending with the start of the P wave of the normal beat following the premature beat. If this distance is the same as the previous one, the pause is a complete compensatory pause. If the start of the P wave on the third beat occurs earlier, the pause is termed an incomplete or non-compensatory pause. Ventricular premature beats are often followed by a complete compensatory pause. This is because atrial depolarization usually occurs as normal. An exception to this are interpolated premature beats, which are ventricular premature beats that occur exactly between two normal sinus beats and don't have any compensatory pause. Atrial premature beats however usually produce incomplete compensatory pauses.

The majority of ventricular premature beats are benign and require no treatment. Patients can be advised to limit alcohol, tobacco and caffeine intake, occasionally beta blockers may be used. There are however some patterns of ventricular premature beat that can lead to more serious arrhythmias, such as VT and VF. These patterns include two or more ventricular premature beats occurring together (Table 6.2).

Most ventricular premature beats are unifocal, occurring from the same place and sharing the same morphology. Sometimes ventricular premature beats can be multifocal and originate from different areas in the ventricle. The presence of multifocal VPBs can indicate serious heart disease. Multifocal VPBs can be identified in the same way as ventricular premature beats with the exception that they differ in morphology from one another (Fig. 6.2).

## Bigeminy and Trigeminy

A regular repeating pattern of premature beats. Bigeminy can be identified by a repeating pattern of normal beat followed by premature beat. Trigeminy is identified by a repeating pattern of premature beat following every two intrinsic beats. Ventricular bigeminy/trigeminy is another pattern of ventricular premature beat that

| **Table 6.2** Pathological patterns of ventricular premature beat | Couplets | 2 ventricular premature beats occurring together |
| --- | --- | --- |
| | Triplets | 3 ventricular premature beats occurring together |
| | Salvos | 4 ventricular premature beats occurring together |

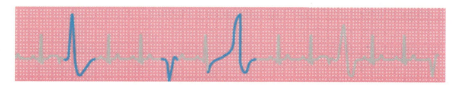

**Fig. 6.2**  Multifocal/multiform ventricular premature beats

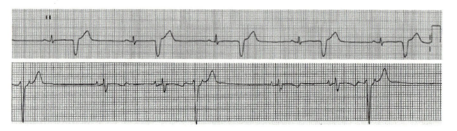

**Fig. 6.3**  (*Top*) Ventricular bigeminy, (*bottom*) ventricular trigeminy

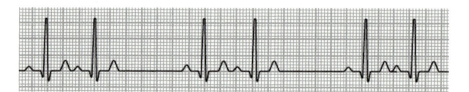

**Fig. 6.4**  Atrial bigeminy

can predispose individuals to dangerous arrhythmias, such as VT/VF. An example of ventricular bigeminy/trigemniny and atrial bigeminy can be seen in Figs. 6.3 and 6.4.

## Supraventricular Tachycardia

Or SVT is a tachycardia that originates from above the ventricles (Fig. 6.5). Therefore SVT is a blanket term for many different forms of tachycardia (Table 6.3). The term SVT is often used when the specific rhythm can not be identified. SVTs usually manifest with rapid narrow QRS complexes, with the caveat of aberrancy, which is discussed later in the chapter.

ST depression and T wave inversion (signs of ischemia) are often associated with SVT. The rate is usually between 100 and 250 BPM. As the electrical impulse travels through the AV node, drugs such as Adenosine can be used to initiate a transient AV block. This can reveal the underlying rhythm making a diagnosis possible. Alternatively the rhythm may be terminated completely if it caused by a reentry pathway that utilizes the AV node. Another option often used to terminate or reveal an underlying rhythm is the use of vagal maneuvers. Some of these maneuvers can even be taught to patients to help them deal with future episodes of SVT.

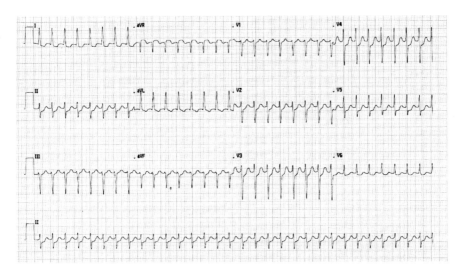

**Fig. 6.5** SVT

**Table 6.3** Types of SVT

| |
| --- |
| Sinus tachycardia |
| Atrial fibrillation |
| Atrial flutter |
| Atrial tachycardia |
| Multifocal atrial tachycardia |
| AV node reentry tachycardia (AVNRT) |
| AV reciprocating tachycardia (AVRT) |

## *Vagal Maneuvers*

The human autonomic nervous system encompasses the sympathetic and parasympathetic divisions. The autonomic nervous system regulates organs and glands at a subconscious level. Stimulating vagal efferent discharge has the effect of inducing transient AV nodal block. This in turn has the effect of terminating tachycardias that subsist on AV conduction, such as AVNRT and AVRT. Other SVTs may be more easily diagnosed by stimulation of the vagus nerve. The vagus nerve can be stimulated by using vagal manoeuvres. Table 6.4 lists some of these vagal manoeuvres.

## Atrial Fibrillation

The single most commonly encountered arrhythmia increases the annual risk of stroke by around 4–5 %. The incidence of Atrial fibrillation (AF) increases with age. AF is also often seen in patients following cardiac surgery.

AF is characterised on the ECG by an irregularly irregular rhythm (Fig. 6.6) best seen in the rhythm strip of an ECG. There is no pattern to the irregularity and a

**Table 6.4** Vagal manoeuvres

| Vagal manoeuvre | Procedure |
|---|---|
| Valsalva | Forced expiration against a closed glottis. This can be done by closing the patients mouth and getting them to pinch their nose. The patient then exhales as if blowing up a balloon. Alternatively a 10 ml syringe may be used. Ask the patient to blow into the tip of the syringe and try to move the plunger. |
| Müeller | Forced inspiration against a closed glottis. Essentially the opposite of the valsalva manoeuvre. |
| Diving reflex | Often used with children. An ice cold bag is applied to the face. This reduces the risk of aspiration associated with submerging the face in ice cold water. |
| Carotid sinus massage | Rotational pressure is applied to the right carotid artery for between 5 and 10 s. Patients should be monitored (including ECG and BP) during procedure. Doctors will often listen for a carotid bruit with a stethoscope as this is a good indicator of carotid arterial stenosis. |
| | Carotid sinus massage is contraindicated in patients with: |
| |    History of TIA or stroke in last 3 months |
| |    Myocardial infarction |
| |    Occlusion of carotid artery |
| |    History of VT or VF |
| |    Previous adverse reaction to sinus massage |
| Ocular pressure | Contraindicated due to the risk of retinal detachment. |
| Coughing | Not technically a manoeuvre but can be used to stimulate the vagal nerve. Encourage the patent to cough hard. |

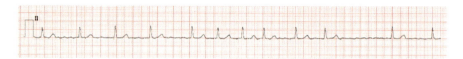

**Fig. 6.6** Atrial fibrillation

chaotic baseline consisting of fibrillatory waves, termed 'f' waves is usually observed. The other salient feature of AF is the complete absence of P waves, best seen in leads II and $V_1$. AF is caused by the presence of multiple ectopic foci in the atria, usually located near the pulmonary veins. These foci act as triggers increasing the atrial rate. The AV node however prevents the majority of impulses being conducted to the ventricles. If this was not the case the outcome would be catastrophic. AF with a ventricular rate <100 BPM is termed 'controlled AF', whereas >100 BPM is referred to as 'uncontrolled' or 'fast' AF. Fibrillation of the atria reduces cardiac output by more than 20 % via loss of 'atrial kick'. The atrial kick is the contribution made by the atria prior to ventricular systole. It has the effect of boosting the efficiency of ventricular ejection.

AF is often detected through manual pulse palpation. When GPs record manual pulses during routine visits leading to the detection of AF, there is a reduction in the incidence of stroke. Unfortunately due the use of technology manual pulse palpation is not being carried out as frequently as it once was. Most machines used to take patients observations do however display the patients pulse. If the pulse is 'jumping around' on the machine in an irregular manner then manual palpation should be carried out. If the pulse appears to be irregular a 12-lead ECG should be carried out.

If the arrhythmia persists, initial electrical remodelling of the atria is subsequently followed by structural remodelling, which in turn helps to maintain the arrhythmia. Atrial remodelling refers to any persisting change in the structure or function of the atria. Atrial remodeling makes it more likely that ectopic or reentry activity will occur. Structural changes induced by AF occur at a cellular level and include many factors, such as: an increase in myocyte cell size, myolysis, changes to the shape of mitochondria, changes to structural proteins and fragmentation of the sarcoplasmic reticulum. Both electrical and structural remodelling maintain the arrhythmia, the longer a patient has AF, the more likely these changes are to occur.

Atrial fibrillation can be further classified as:

- Paroxysmal Atrial Fibrillation
    Terminates spontaneously, usually in less than 7 days
- Persistent Atrial Fibrillation
    Does not terminate spontaneously and lasts longer than 7 days
- Permanent Atrial Fibrillation
    Not terminated or reverted.

Patients presenting with AF who have been in fibrillation for longer than 48 h require anticoagulation prior to direct current cardioversion (DCCV). This is due to the possibility that intramural thrombus may accumulate in the atria, often around the left atrial appendage. When the normal motion of the atrium is recommenced, there is a risk that the thrombus may migrate causing a stroke. To mitigate against this anticoagulation is given for weeks before and after the cardioversion. If this is not possible due to hemodynamic compromise requiring immediate treatment, IV heparin can be administered prior to the cardioversion.

Patients with a prior history of AF suffering a new incidence of AF for less than 48 h can suffer from remodelling of the atria caused by the previous episodes of AF. In this case there may be an increased risk involved in DCCV. To be sure that there are no intramural thrombi present the patient may have a transoesophageal echocardiogram (TOE). This involves passing an ultrasound sensor into the oesophagus to better view the chambers of the heart.

Treatment for AF focuses on either rate control or rhythm control. Rate control aims to reduce symptoms associated with the high heart rates and to prevent cardiomyopathy secondary to the tachycardia. Rhythm control on the other hand aims to terminate the underlying rhythm. Generally paroxysmal AF is treated initially with rhythm control. Permanent AF alternatively is usually treated with rate control strategies. Persistent AF can be treated with either. In these patients rhythm control is often tried first if they are younger, symptomatic or have congestive heart failure. Rate control is attempted first in older patients (>65 years), unsuitable for cardioversion or treatment with antiarrhythmic drugs or with coronary artery disease. If either of the options attempted first fails the patient may be considered for the alternative strategy. Figures 6.7 and 6.8 show the treatment algorithms recommended by NICE

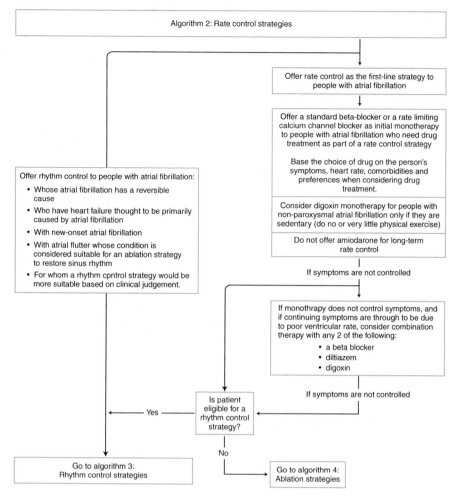

**Fig. 6.7** Rate control strategies adapted from NICE, (2014) guidelines on the management of AF

in their management of atrial fibrillation guidelines for both rhythm and rate control (2014). The symptoms and causes of AF are listed in Tables 6.5 and 6.6.

Rhythm control options include:

- Direct current cardioversion
- Chemical/pharmacological cardioversion
- Ablation
- Cox maze surgical procedure (deliberate scarring of the atrium to block atrial macroreentry)

Rate control options focus on treatment with medication to reduced the rate. They include:

- Beta Blockers with calcium channel blockers
- Digoxin

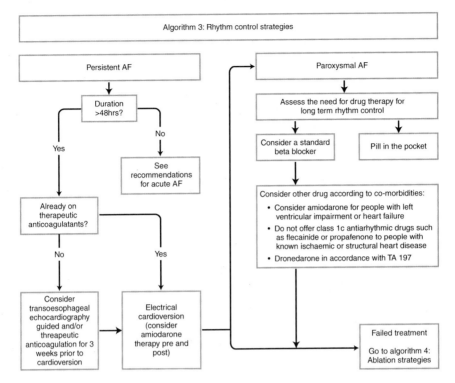

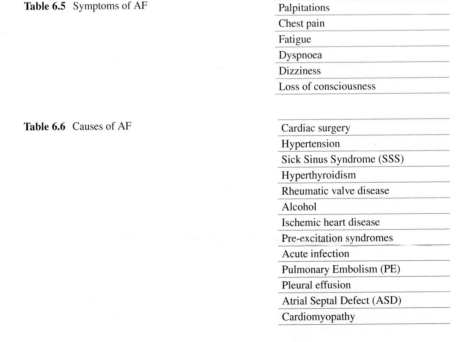

**Fig. 6.8** Rhythm control strategies adapted from NICE, (2014) guidelines on the management of AF

**Table 6.5** Symptoms of AF

| Palpitations |
| --- |
| Chest pain |
| Fatigue |
| Dyspnoea |
| Dizziness |
| Loss of consciousness |

**Table 6.6** Causes of AF

| Cardiac surgery |
| --- |
| Hypertension |
| Sick Sinus Syndrome (SSS) |
| Hyperthyroidism |
| Rheumatic valve disease |
| Alcohol |
| Ischemic heart disease |
| Pre-excitation syndromes |
| Acute infection |
| Pulmonary Embolism (PE) |
| Pleural effusion |
| Atrial Septal Defect (ASD) |
| Cardiomyopathy |

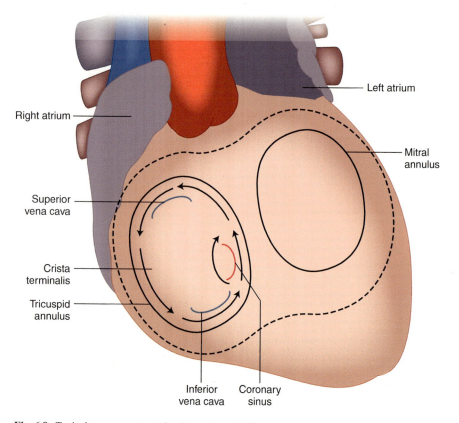

**Fig. 6.9**  Typical macroreentrant circuit seen in atrial flutter

## Atrial Flutter

Is caused by a macroreentrant circuit and is usually paroxysmal. Atrial flutter usually originates from the right atrium. Atrial flutter and atrial fibrillation are closely linked and may alternate in individuals. The symptoms and causes of atrial flutter are the same as those for AF. A prolonged atrial flutter often converts itself into atrial fibrillation. Figure 6.9 shows a typical macroreentrant circuit seen in the right atrium, the arrows show the direction the pathway sustaining the flutter. The AV node cannot conduct impulses at these high rates to the ventricles as a degree of heart block develops.

Flutter can be identified on the ECG by its classic 'sawtooth' like appearance, seen best in lead II, III and aVF. As with Atrial Fibrillation there are no P waves, but instead prominent Flutter 'F' waves (Fig. 6.10). It is also worth noting that flutter waves in lead $V_1$ can look like P waves. The atrial rate of atrial flutter is often around 300 and usually between 200 and 400 impulses per minute.

There are different conduction ratios between the atrial and ventricular rates. These ratios usually remain the same but can sometimes manifest with a variable AV block. The term AV block when used in relation to atrial flutter is not the same

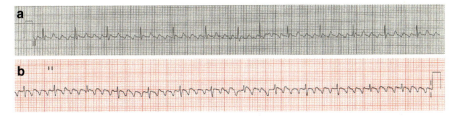

**Fig. 6.10** Atrial flutter seen in lead II rhythm strip

**Table 6.7** Degree of block related to heart rate based on flutter wave rate of 300 BPM

| Heart rate (BPM) | Degree of block |
|---|---|
| 150 | 2:1 |
| 100 | 3:1 |
| 75 | 4:1 |

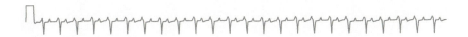

**Fig. 6.11** Atrial tachycardia

thing as AV block in terms of heart block as the AV node is functioning normally in flutter, it is just responding to rapid atrial rates by being unable to conduct all the atrial impulses due to refractory periods.

Atrial flutter should be considered when presented with any SVT at a rate of 150 BPM. This could well be an atrial flutter with a 2:1 block. Vagal manoeuvres or Adenosine can be potentially used to reveal the underlying rhythm as discussed previously. Common degrees of block relating to the heart rate can be seen in Table 6.7.

There are two primary types of atrial flutter, type I and type II. Type I flutter is also referred to as typical or common atrial flutter. There are two further subdivision of type I atrial flutter; clockwise and counterclockwise type I atrial flutter.

The reentry pathway usually takes an counterclockwise direction as seen in Fig. 6.9. and can be differentiated from clockwise flutter on the ECG by inverted flutter waves in the inferior leads II, III and aVF. Clockwise flutter on the other hand is the exact opposite (upright in II, III and aVF). Type II atrial flutter, also called uncommon or atypical atrial flutter is more difficult to identify. It usually occurs at higher atrial rates (340–440 BPM) and does not fulfil the criteria of typical atrial flutter.

# Atrial Tachycardia

Is characterized by the presence of three or more atrial premature beats, and an atrial rate of between 140 and 250 BPM (Fig. 6.11). P waves, best seen in leads II or $V_1$ are sometime present and usually hidden in the preceding T waves. The rhythm is regular. Atrial Tachycardia can also cause loss of 'atrial kick' and a reduced cardiac output if sustained.

**Table 6.8**  Causes of atrial tachycardia

| |
| --- |
| Caffeine and other stimulants |
| Physical/emotional stress |
| Hypoxia |
| Electrolyte imbalance |
| Cardiomyopathy |
| MI |

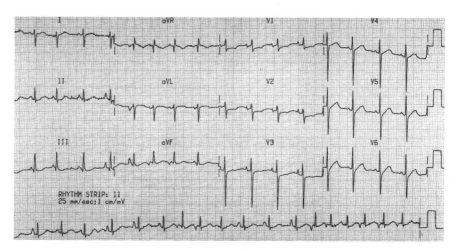

**Fig. 6.12**  MAT [Life in the Fast Lane   (http://lifeinthefastlane.com/education/procedures/lead-positioning/)/CC BY-SA 4.0 (http://creativecommons.org/licenses/by-sa/4.0/)]

The tachycardia usually originates from an ectopic foci inside the atrium but not from the sinoatrial node. The arrhythmia is usually sustained by an atrial reentry circuit. The P waves, if they can be seen usually have a different morphology to the patients normal P wave. Atrial tachycardia is rarely sustained and is usually paroxysmal. Table 6.8 shows causes of atrial tachycardia.

## Multifocal Atrial Tachycardia

Or MAT as it is sometimes referred is quite rare and is therefore possibly under-diagnosed. It may often be mistaken for AF as it also manifests with an irregularly irregular rhythm at a ventricular rate >100 BPM. There are however P waves present, but as they are due to three or more ectopic foci the P wave morphologies will vary from one another (Fig. 6.12). MAT tends to occur in very ill individuals with severe infection and/or respiratory failure, such as COPD and CHF. It can also be caused by hypoxia, severe pulmonary disease, atrial dysfunction or ischemic heart disease. MAT carries a poor prognosis, with death occurring usually as a result of the underlying condition rather than the arrhythmia. As such MAT tends to be

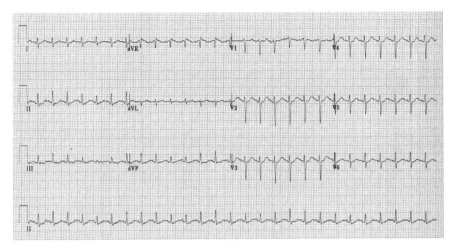

**Fig. 6.13** Sinus tachycardia [Life in the Fast Lane (http://lifeinthefastlane.com/education/proce-dures/lead-positioning/)/CC BY-SA 4.0 (http://creativecommons.org/licenses/by-sa/4.0/)]

| **Table 6.9** Causes of sinus tachycardia | |
| --- | --- |
| | Overstimulation of the sympathetic nervous system |
| | Anxiety/pain |
| | PE |
| | Pericarditis |
| | Anaemia |
| | Heart failure |
| | Pregnancy |
| | Stimulants |
| | Infection |
| | hyperthyroidism |
| | Hypotension |

mostly seen in intensive care or high dependency units. A multifocal atrial tachycar-dia with a rate <100 BPM is referred to as wandering atrial pacemaker and is caused by other pacemaker sites in the atria or junctional region temporarily taking over due to increased vagal tone.

## Sinus Tachycardia

A sinus rhythm with a rate greater than 100 BPM is defined as a sinus tachycardia (Fig. 6.13). Sinus tachycardia may result from infection, use of stimulants, such as tobacco and caffeine and various other medical conditions summarised in Table 6.9.

## Sinus Arrhythmia

The presence of normal intrinsic PQRST waves but with an irregular rhythm (Fig. 6.14). A 10 % variance in the P to P cycle (the distance between two consecutive P waves) is considered normal. A variation above 10 % points towards sinus arrhythmia. The rhythm is essentially caused by irregular rates of sinus node impulse generation. The rhythm usually causes no symptoms and requires no treatment. If treatment is required then Atropine or exercise are often used to terminate the arrhythmia.

The rhythm is also linked to the respiratory cycle with inspiration reducing the P-P cycle increasing the heart rate. Sinus arrhythmia can be caused or seen in patients with: diabetes, alcoholic cardiomyopathy, raised intracranial pressure and those taking Digoxin.

## Junctional Tachycardia

A tachycardia can also originate from the junctional region (Fig. 6.15). P waves when visible are often seen after the QRS complex and activate the atria retrogradely.

### *Reentry*

Is triggered by an impulse returning to depolarize previously depolarized tissue a second time. For this to occur there needs to be a triggering stimulus and a potential reentry pathway. Patients with ischemic disease or congenital accessory pathways are prone to arrhythmias.

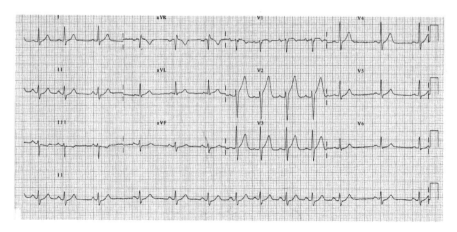

**Fig. 6.14** Sinus arrhythmia [Life in the Fast Lane  (http://lifeinthefastlane.com/education/procedures/lead-positioning/)/CC BY-SA 4.0 (http://creativecommons.org/licenses/by-sa/4.0/)]

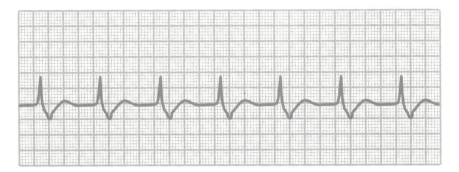

**Fig. 6.15** Junctional tachycardia

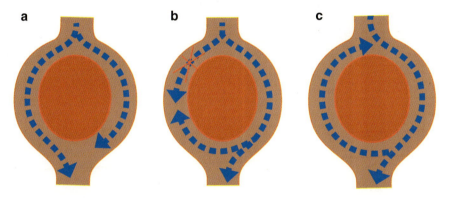

**Fig. 6.16** Arrhythmogenic mechanisms

A premature beat can initiate a tachycardia in patients with a reentry circuit. Sometimes the impulse can travel down both limbs of a circuit (Fig. 6.16a). Alternatively one limb of a ring of cardiac tissue is more refractory than the other the impulse then proceeds slowly down the pathway and then back up through the once blocked section (Fig. 6.16b). Finally the impulse can travel very slowly along one pathway and then backtrack back through the other limb (Fig. 6.16c).

There are several types of reentry circuits that can trigger a supraventricular tachycardia, these include:

- SA nodal reentry
- AV nodal reentry
- AV nodal bypass reentry

SA nodal reentry is classified as a macroreentrant tachycardia and occurs within the sinoatrial node itself (Fig. 6.17). These fast and slow pathways can also exist in the AV node (Fig. 6.18) and is referred to as AV nodal reentry tachycardia (AVNRT). AVNRT is also the most commonly encountered. AVNRT is seen on the ECG as

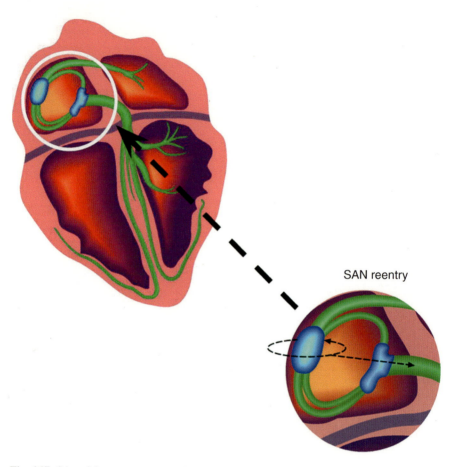

SAN reentry

**Fig. 6.17** SA nodal reentry

regular, fast rhythm with a rate usually above 130 BPM. Retrograde P waves are also often present, appearing at the end of the QRS complexes. A small secondary R wave similar to the one seen in RBBB but without the widened QRS is also often seen, as is a RP interval of <100 ms. The other mechanism for reentry is an extra pathway that bypasses the AV node entirely allowing impulses to go back up through this pathway creating a sustained loop (Fig. 6.18).

## Pre-excitation

Refers to the activation of the ventricles by a congenital accessory pathway. Wolff-Parkinson-White syndrome is an example of pre-excitation.

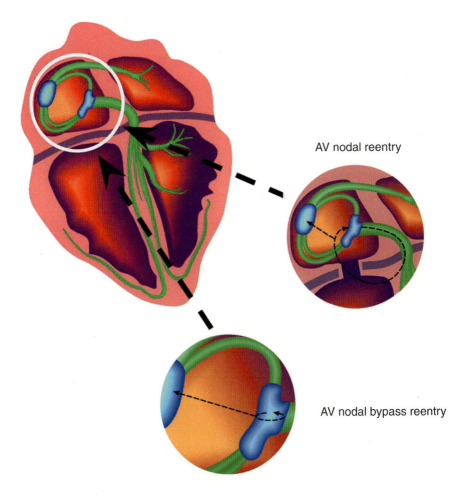

AV nodal reentry

AV nodal bypass reentry

**Fig. 6.18** AV nodal reentry

## Wolff-Parkinson-White Syndrome (WPW)

Is the most common form pre-excitation and was named after its discoverers. A foetal abnormality results in a pathway that connects the atria and ventricles. The atria and ventricles are electrically isolated by the atrioventricular ring, allowing impulses to only travel between atria and ventricles by the conduction pathway. This extra pathway is referred to as the bundle of Kent and allows impulses to travel via the bundle. Impulses can also travel back up to the atria from the ventricles creating a sustained tachycardia. WPW normally occurs in the young and adults aged 20–35 years of age. Most people with this condition seek medical attention due to the frequent occurrence of supraventricular tachyarrhythmias. Because there is no AV node to slow the impulse in the accessory pathway the PR

**Fig. 6.19** The delta wave
and short PR interval
associated with WPW

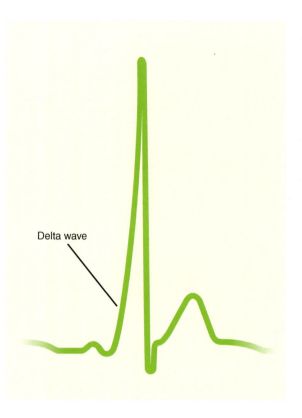

Delta wave

interval is short. The impulse is then slower to activate the ventricles as it is not passing through the normal conduction system. This leads to the formation of a 'delta wave' on the ECG. The short PR interval and delta wave are the key ECG features of this syndrome. Figures 6.19 and 6.20 shows the slurred upstroke termed a delta wave and short PR interval with the P wave located very closely to the QRS complex.

There are two subtypes of WPW called type A and type B WPW. These subtypes can be identified by looking at the deflection of QRS complexes in $V_1$.

- Type A – QRS complexes are positively deflected in $V_1$
- Type B – QRS complexes are negatively deflected in $V_1$

## *Orthodromic and Antidromic*

The direction the impulse takes through the accessory pathway is referred to as orthodromic or antidromic and can distinguished on the ECG by broad or narrow QRS complexes (Table 6.10).

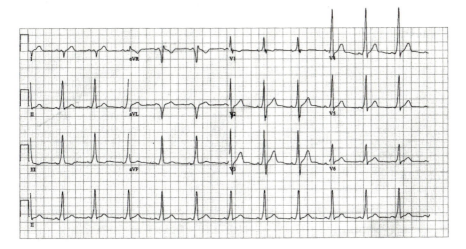

**Fig. 6.20** WPW (type A)

**Table 6.10** Orthodromic and antidromic

| Orthodromic | Antidromic |
|---|---|
| 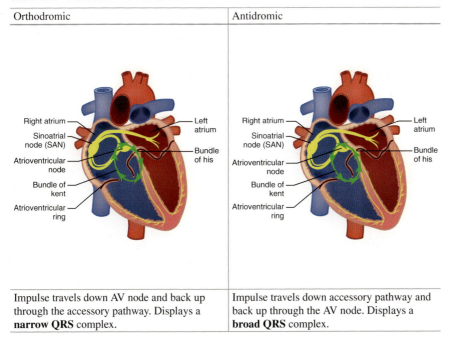 | |
| Impulse travels down AV node and back up through the accessory pathway. Displays a **narrow QRS** complex. | Impulse travels down accessory pathway and back up through the AV node. Displays a **broad QRS** complex. |

## *Wolff-Parkinson-White Syndrome and Atrial Fibrillation*

Atrial fibrillation or less commonly flutter can occur in patients with WPW (Fig. 6.21). The accessory pathway allows impulses to bypass the AV node and

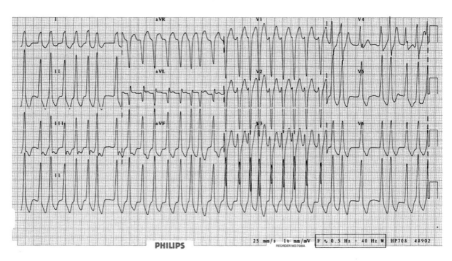

**Fig. 6.21** WPW and AF [Life in the Fast Lane (http://lifeinthefastlane.com/education/procedures/lead-positioning/)/CC BY-SA 4.0 (http://creativecommons.org/licenses/by-sa/4.0/)]

| **Table 6.11** Contraindicated drugs for treatment of WPW and AF | IV Adenosine |
| --- | --- |
| | Verapamil |
| | Digoxin |
| | Diltiazem |

conduct the ventricles rapidly. There is also a possibility the rhythm will degenerate to VT or VF. Adenosine is contraindicated in WPW with atrial fibrillation as it may lead to 1:1 conduction. Other drugs that should not be administered are shown in Table 6.11. DC cardioversion is however safe and effective.

## Lown-Ganong-Levine Syndrome (LGL)

More common in the young and women, patients also present with tachyarrhythmias. Like WPW it was also named after the people who discovered the syndrome. The main ECG findings are a short PR interval, no delta wave and episodes of reentrant tachycardia (Fig. 6.22). The exact mechanisms precipitating this syndrome are not fully understood. Some experts believed in the past that accessory pathways, such as James fibres or Brechenmacher fibres allowed impulses to bypass all or part of the AV node. Enhanced AV nodal conduction is now considered to be the primary mechanism. Electrophysiological studies have shown that there are often different arrhythmic mechanisms at work in so called LGL syndrome and that the label of LGL is used to describe a short PR interval with normal but accelerated AV nodal conduction caused by various different arrhythmogenic mechanisms.

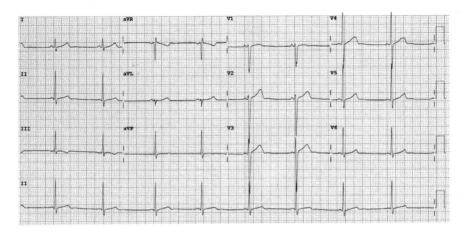

**Fig. 6.22** LGL syndrome

## Cardioversion

Direct current cardioversion (DCCV) is used when an arrhythmia leads to haemo-dynamic compromise or for routine planned cardioversion of an arrhythmia. If the patient has no cardiac output then unsynchronised defibrillation is carried out.

DCCV is used to treat cardiac arrhythmias by depolarizing the cells of the myocardium. This is done via an electrical current delivered through defibrillator pads applied to the patient. It is hoped that following depolarization of the heart, normal repolarization will occur and the cardiac arrhythmia will be terminated.

Synchronised cardioversion can be used if R waves are visible on the ECG. Modern defibrillators have the ability to synchronize the electrical discharge 20 ms (0.02 s) after the R wave. This is done to apply the current to the myocardium at a point when the cells are in a state of depolarization. If the current were to be discharged during the relative refractory period (Fig. 6.23) it could trigger 'R on T' phenomenon, which can precipitate VF and polymorphic VT. The relative risks and benefits of DCCV can be seen Table 6.12.

## Electrophysiology Studies (EPS)

Catheters can be placed in the heart via a vein or artery (Fig. 6.24), usually in the groin. The catheters are placed by x-ray. The procedure allows detailed examination of the heart's electrical system to be carried out. Electrodes can also be used to pace the heart to stimulate arrhythmias so the source can be detected.

**Fig. 6.23** Synchronized cardioversion

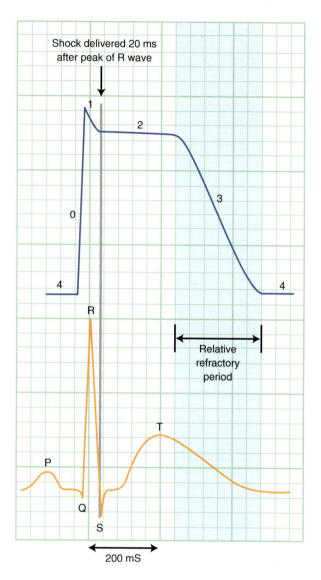

**Table 6.12** Risks and benefits of DCCV

| Risks | Benefits |
|---|---|
| Thromboembolism | Successful when pharmacological cardioversion does not work |
| Anaesthetic complications | Immediate arrhythmia cessation |
| Cardiac arrest VT/VF | Reduction of side effects associated with antiarrhythmic drugs |
| Burns/thoracic pain | |

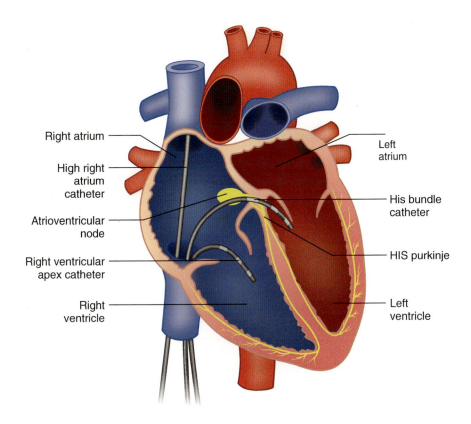

**Fig. 6.24** Conventional catheter placement sites for EPS

## *Ablation*

Once the source of the arrhythmia has been located ablation may be offered. Ablation is a method of destroying cells that are supporting an arrhythmia. Radiofrequency ablation is often used to burn cells. Cryoablation is also utilized in some centres and allows cells to be destroyed using extreme cold. The advantage of cryotherapy is that cells can be frozen to see their effect on the arrhythmia before they are permanently destroyed. If the wrong cells are targeted they can potentially recover.

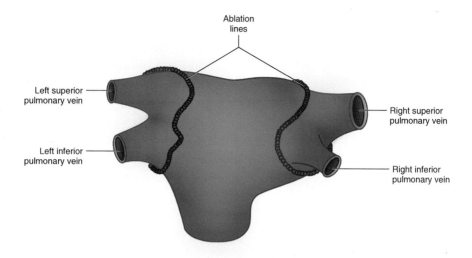

**Fig. 6.25** Electroanatomic mapping

As mentioned previously the ectopic foci in AF are usually sited around the pulmonary veins. Ablation can be used as a treatment option for AF. Some electrophysiologists use 3D electroanatomic mapping systems (Fig. 6.25) to map the intended ablation sites. Ablation of ectopic foci around the pulmonary veins is >90 % effective for treating AF, however there is good chance the AF will return within the first year following treatment (30–50 %).

Another option is to use ablation to deliberately destroy the patients AV junction. This creates a complete conduction block preventing rapid ventricular activation. The patient then has a permanent pacemaker implanted and becomes totally pacemaker dependent. To reduce the need for temporary pacing prior to permanent pacemaker insertion, a pacemaker may be implanted several weeks before the ablation. Figure 6.26 displays the NICE algorithm for left atrial ablation.

It is also often possible to use ablation to treat atrial flutter. This is done by scarring tissue in the path of the circuit causing the flutter.

## Ventricular Tachycardia (VT)

VT is a broad complex tachycardia with a rate $\geq$120 BPM. Four or more ventricular premature beats constitutes a run of VT. Sustained VT is defined as VT that lasts for more than 30 s. It can be challenging to differentiate between a ventricular tachycardia and a supraventricular tachycardia with aberration.

Aberrant conduction is essentially conduction of an impulse from supraventricular region to the ventricles in a significantly different way from normal conduction.

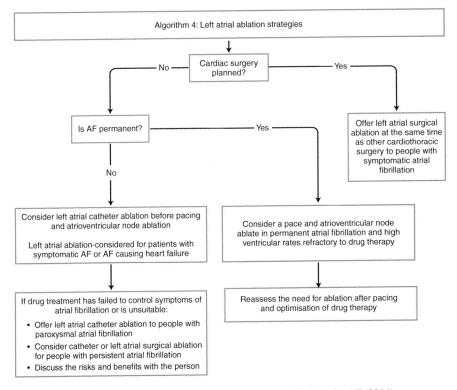

**Fig. 6.26** Ablation strategies algorithm adapted from NICE guidelines for AF (2014)

This is especially possible in patients with a bundle branch block or WPW syndrome. If the rate is rapid and the aberrant conduction causes the appearance of wide QRS complexes, an SVT can look like a VT. Distinguishing between the two can be very important as AV blocking agents that work well for terminating SVT can cause haemodynamic instability if given to a patient with VT. Fortunately DC cardioversion is a safe and effective option for both VT and SVT.

Telling the difference between VT and SVT with aberrancy can be done by systematic examination to look for supporting evidence of a ventricular tachycardia. The more evidence the more likely it is to be a VT. Firstly VT is more commonly encountered than SVT with aberrancy. Clues to the presence of ventricular ectopy include:

## *Fusion Beats*

Caused by impulses from different locations occurring simultaneously in the same region of the heart (Fig. 6.27). The beat can literally look like the merging of two different beats together.

**Fig. 6.27**  A fusion beat
(*BMJ* 2002)

**Figure 6.28**  A capture beat
(*BMJ* 2002)

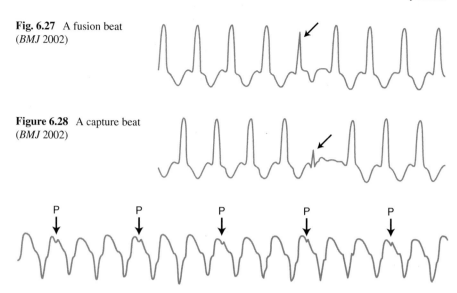

**Fig. 6.29**  AV dissociation (P waves indicated by *arrows*)

## Capture Beats

Are caused by temporary reassertion of the SA node over the ventricles leading to a subsequent QRS complex of normal duration (Fig. 6.28).

## AV Dissociation

Regularly occurring P waves may be seen on the ECG but have no relationship to the QRS complexes (Fig. 6.29) increasing the likelihood of the rhythm being VT.

## Rhythm Regularity

If the rhythm is markedly irregularly irregular it may suggest atrial fibrillation which would make it probable that it was a SVT not a VT. Some small irregularity is also common in VT.

## Concordance

Refers to the deflection of complexes in leads $V_1$ to $V_6$ being the same. If they are predominantly deflected in the same direction then concordance exists and provides additional evidence for the presence of VT. If there is no concordance however it could still be VT. Concordance can be either positive or negative.

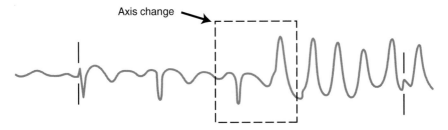

**Fig. 6.30** A change of QRS axis (deflected in opposite direction to normal sinus rhythm)

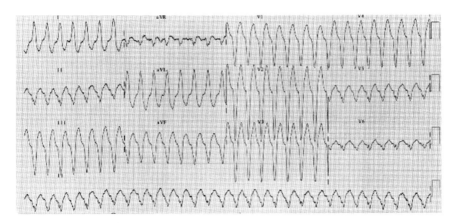

**Fig. 6.31** A monomorphic VT

## *Cardiac Axis*

The QRS axis will be different to the axis of the normal sinus rhythm (Fig. 6.30). This also favors a VT diagnosis.

There are several subtypes of VT, including:

- Monomorphic/unifocal VT
  - Right ventricular outflow tract VT (RVOT)
  - Fascicular VT
- Polymorphic VT

Monomorphic VT is a form of VT where the beats share the same morphology (they look the same). This is because the source of ectopic focus is the same (Fig. 6.31).

A form of monomorphic VT called Right ventricular outflow tract tachycardia (RVOT) that originates from the right ventricular outflow tract. RVOT is a tachycardia that has LBBB morphology with rightward axis of around +90° (Fig. 6.32). The condition is often seen in patients with Arrhythmogenic Right Ventricular Dysplasia/ Cardiomyopathy (ARVD/C).

Fascicular tachycardia is another monomorphic VT that is characterised by a RBBB pattern with axis deviation (Table 6.13). Fascicular tachycardia originates from the posterior or anterior fascicle of the left bundle branch.

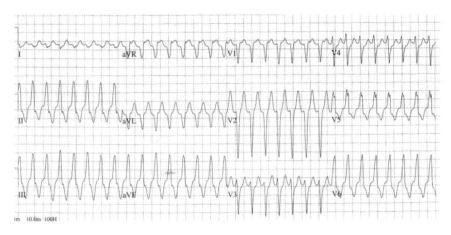

**Fig. 6.32** Right ventricular outflow tract tachycardia (RVOT)

| Table 6.13 Defining ECG features of posterior and anterior fascicular VT | Fascicle | Details |
|---|---|---|
| | Posterior | RBBB pattern with left axis deviation |
| | Anterior | RBBB pattern with right axis deviation |

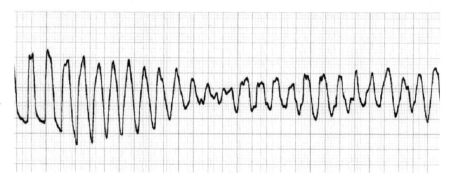

**Fig. 6.33** Torsades de pointes

Polymorphic VT is a form of VT where there are multiple ventricular ectopic foci. Polymorphic VT is often seen in the context of myocardial infarction. The axis and amplitude of the QRS complexes vary. Torsades de pointes is a French name for twisting about points (Fig. 6.33). This is a type of polymorphic VT that is associated with a long QT interval unlike other forms of polymorphic VT which occur with a normal QT interval.

Idioventricular rhythm is also referred to as slow VT and is a reperfusion arrhythmia associated with myocardial infarction. Idioventricular rhythm is discussed in more detail in Chap. 7.

**Fig. 6.34** Chest compressions

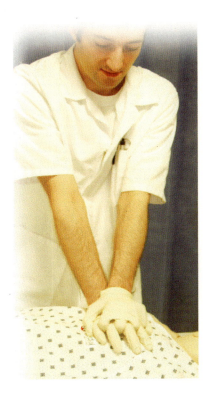

## Cardiac Arrest Rhythms

A cardiac arrest occurs when the heart fails to pump enough blood around the body to sustain life. Loss of consciousness occurs due to lack of oxygen and glucose to the brain. A cardiac arrest is a medical emergency and requires immediate intervention to prevent death. Prompt CPR and defibrillation (if the rhythm is shockable) should be applied as soon as possible. Delays in receiving prompt treatment can lead to death or a degree of brain damage. Chest compressions (Fig. 6.34) provided by cardiopulmonary resuscitation (CPR) are instrumental in providing a flow of oxygenated blood to the brain and other organs delaying permanent tissue death. There are certain causes of cardiac arrest that have the potential to be treated and terminate the arrest. These factors are referred to as the reversible causes and are summarised in Table 6.14. Attempts to identify these causes should be made whilst providing immediate/advanced life support. The principle cardiac arrest rhythms comprise of:

- Pulseless ventricular tachycardia
- Ventricular fibrillation
- Asystole
- Pulseless electrical activity

| **Table 6.14** The potentially reversible causes of cardiac arrest | Hypoxia |
| --- | --- |
| | Hypovolaemia |
| | Hypo/hyperkalemia and other metabolic |
| | Hypothermia |
| | Tension pneumothorax |
| | Tamponade |
| | Toxins |
| | Thrombosis (either cardiac or pulmonary) |

**Fig. 6.35** Ventricular flutter

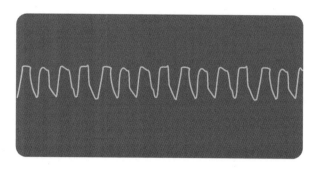

Of the four primary arrest rhythms, only VF and VT are 'shockable' rhythms (respond favorably to defibrillation). Both VT and VF have better outcomes than the other arrest rhythms.

## Pulseless VT

The same as VT but sustained and not producing sufficient cardiac output to generate a pulse. In this case defibrillation is used to attempt to restore sinus rhythm.

## Ventricular Flutter

A form of VT with a very rapid rate (250–350 BPM) presenting with a monomorphic sine wave like appearance (Fig. 6.35). Ventricular flutter normally rapidly progresses to ventricular fibrillation.

## Ventricular Fibrillation

Rapid irregular electrical activity producing no cardiac output. There are no discernable waveforms or intervals. VF can appear coarse or fine (Fig. 6.36). Fine VF follows coarse VF and reduces the chance of successful treatment as myocardial

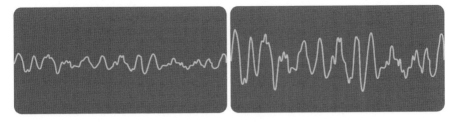

**Fig. 6.36** (*Left*) fine VF,
(*right*) coarse (VF)

**Fig. 6.37** Asystole

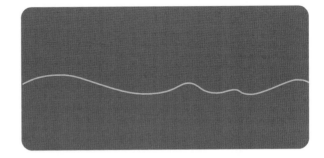

metabolic energy stores are further depleted resulting eventually in asystole. Sometimes VF can be so fine that it can be mistaken for asystole. Increasing the gain on the monitor is one way of revealing any hidden VF rhythm.

## Asystole

Absence of any ventricular or atrial activity (Fig. 6.37). There is no cardiac output in this rhythm and unless reversible causes are present the outlook is extremely poor. Sometimes P waves may be present (termed P wave asystole), these patients may be suitable for pacing. It is also important to check the gain on the monitor as fine VF can sometimes be missed as it can look like asystole if not set properly (1 mV per cm). A complete flat line on a monitor is an indication that one of the monitoring leads may not be connected properly.

## Pulseless Electrical Activity

Used to be called electromechanical dissociation. Essentially coordinated electrical impulse generation is taking place but there is no cardiac output. This is another reason to remember the old adage about treating the patient not the rhythm. The patient will be unconscious and not breathing but a rhythm that should produce a pulse is seen on the monitor. Defibrillation is not appropriate as the issue is caused by lack of response to electrical impulses rather than the impulses themselves.

## Summary of Key Points

- Atrial fibrillation is the most commonly encountered cardiac arrhythmia
- There are various patterns of premature ventricular beats that can predispose individuals to dangerous arrhythmias such as VT and VF
- SVT is a blanket term for arrhythmias occurring above the ventricles
- VT and VF are the only arrest rhythms thats respond to defibrillation
- Cardioversion is a safe and effective treatment for both SVT and VT
- Torsades de pointes is a polymorphic VT that can only be diagnosed in patients with QT prolongation
- An SVT with a regular rate of 150 BPM may be atrial flutter
- Vagal manoeuvres or Adenosine can be potentially used to reveal an arrhythmia in patients with SVT

## Quiz

Q1. Occasional ventricular premature beats

(A) Should be treated as a medical emergency
(B) Do not usually require any treatment
(C) Always require monitoring

Q2. An irregularly irregular rhythm with no P waves is

(A) Atrial flutter
(B) Atrial bigeminy
(C) Atrial fibrillation

Q3. An SVT with a rate of 150 BPM could be

(A) Atrial flutter
(B) WPW
(C) Multifocal atrial tachycardia

Q4. When unsure if a tachycardia is ventricular or supraventricular in origin you should

(A) Use Adenosine
(B) Use electrical cardioversion
(C) Use Digoxin

Q5. A sudden axis change from the normal rhythm in a tachycardia favours VT

(A) True
(B) False

Q6. The main mechanisms of arrhythmogenesis are

    (A) Triggered activity, abnormal/enhanced automaticity and reentry
    (B) Triggered activity, abnormal/enhanced automaticity and bigeminy
    (C) Activated activity, ventricular automaticity and junctional reentry

Interpret the following ECGs

**Q7.**

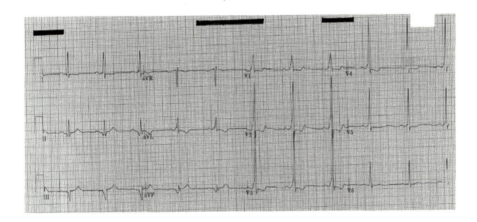

**Q8.**

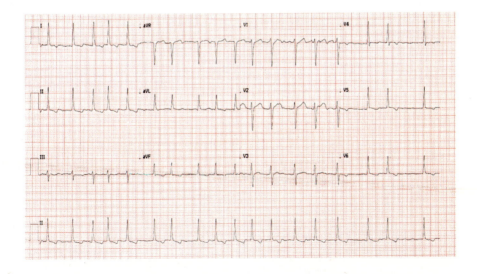

**Q9.**

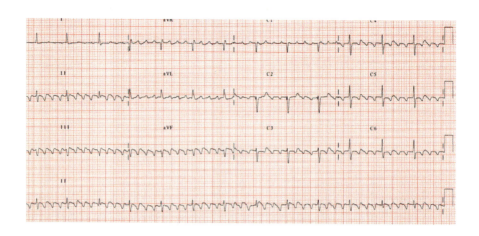

**Q10.**

Answers:  Q1 = B,  Q2 = C,  Q3 = A,  Q4 = B,  Q5 = A,  Q6 = A,  Q7 = WPW,  Q8 = AF,
Q9 = Atrial flutter,  Q10 = Ventricular trigeminy

# Chapter 7
# Acute Coronary Syndromes

**Keywords** ACS • STEMI • NSTEMI • Angina • ST elevation • ST depression • Myocardial infarction • Biomarkers • Reciprocal changes

## Background

Acute coronary syndromes are a group of conditions precipitated by a reduction or cessation of blood flow through the coronary arteries. An acute coronary syndrome (ACS) is a medical emergency requiring immediate intervention. ACS encompasses any narrowing or obstruction of the coronary arteries leading to acute symptoms. Acute coronary syndromes include:

- ST elevation myocardial infarction (STEMI)
- Non ST elevation myocardial infarction (NSTEMI)
- Unstable angina

To better understand these syndromes it is necessary to gain an awareness of how the coronary arteries function and their anatomy. There a two principle coronary arteries, the left and right coronary arteries (Fig. 7.1). The left further subdivides into the left anterior descending and circumflex arteries that supply blood to the left side and front of the heart. The right coronary artery divides into the posterior descending and acute marginal arteries, supplying blood to the right atrium, right ventricle, SAN and AV node and some part of the left ventricle (Fig. 7.2).

The coronary arteries arise from the aorta and supply the heart muscle with blood and oxygen. The artery that supplies the posterior descending artery and one or more posterolateral branches is referred to as the dominant vessel. The right coronary artery is the dominant vessel in 80–85 % of cases, other people have a left dominant or codominant systems.

Any narrowing or blockage to these arteries can reduce or prevent blood flow reaching portions of the heart past the area of narrowing or blockage, leading in turn to an acute coronary syndrome. ACS often presents as chest pain, or tightness/discomfort of the chest. Pain may be accompanied by sweating and nausea. The pain

© Springer-Verlag London 2015
A. Davies, A. Scott, *Starting to Read ECGs: A Comprehensive Guide to Theory and Practice*, DOI 10.1007/978-1-4471-4965-1_7

**Fig. 7.1** The coronary arteries

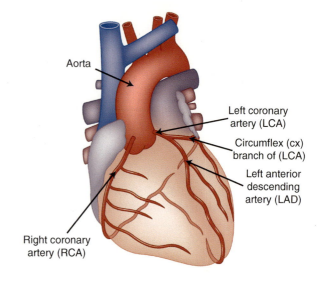

Aorta

Left coronary artery (LCA)

Circumflex (cx) branch of (LCA)

Left anterior descending artery (LAD)

Right coronary artery (RCA)

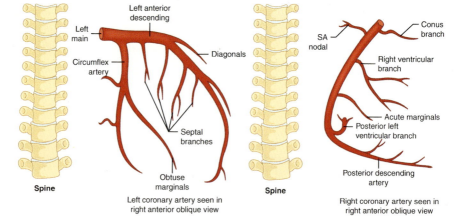

Left anterior descending

Left main

Circumflex artery

Diagonals

Septal branches

Obtuse marginals

**Spine**

Left coronary artery seen in right anterior oblique view

SA nodal

Conus branch

Right ventricular branch

Acute marginals
Posterior left ventricular branch

Posterior descending artery

**Spine**

Right coronary artery seen in right anterior oblique view

**Fig. 7.2**   Left and right coronary artery anatomy

may spread to other areas including the back, shoulders, neck, jaw and arms. The reason pain is felt in areas other than the chest, such as the arm and jaw is due to the brain's inability to distinguish between visceral and somatic sensory distribution. Somatic pain originates in deep tissues and skin, whereas visceral pain derives from internal organs. This confusion originates from the fact that the visceral and somatic nerves from the heart and spinal nerves enter the spinal cord at the same point, causing the brain to interpret the pain as originating from the somatic regions. When a patient presents with chest pain it is important to rule out any other causes (Table 7.1) and ask appropriate questions to ascertain the type of pain the patient is experiencing

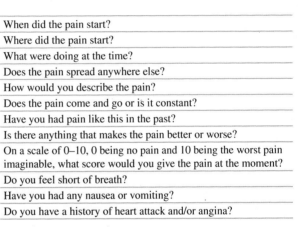

**Table 7.1** Chest pain differential diagnosis

| Pericarditis/myocarditis |
| Tamponade |
| Angina |
| Dissecting aortic aneurysm |
| Oesophageal pain |
| Musculoskeletal pain |
| Pulmonary embolism |
| Trauma |
| Panic attack |
| Arrhythmia |
| Pleurisy |
| Mastitis (seen in breastfeeding women) |

**Table 7.2** Chest pain history questions

| When did the pain start? |
| Where did the pain start? |
| What were doing at the time? |
| Does the pain spread anywhere else? |
| How would you describe the pain? |
| Does the pain come and go or is it constant? |
| Have you had pain like this in the past? |
| Is there anything that makes the pain better or worse? |
| On a scale of 0–10, 0 being no pain and 10 being the worst pain imaginable, what score would you give the pain at the moment? |
| Do you feel short of breath? |
| Have you had any nausea or vomiting? |
| Do you have a history of heart attack and/or angina? |

(Table 7.2) and if it is cardiac in origin. Patients presenting with acute chest pain suspect of ACS should have the following assessments carried out:

- 12-lead ECG on admission followed by serial ECGs as required
- Haemodynamic assessment
- Complete medical history and history of presenting complaint
- Blood test for cardiac biochemical markers

Suspected MI patients should have access to defibrillation, high flow oxygen and analgesia, usually an opiate given with an antiemetic. Cyclizine is not recommended due its potential hemodynamic effects. Antiplatelet aggregators, such as Aspirin are often given to impair platelet aggregation around the clot. Low molecular weight heparins are also often used in ACS patients to reduce coagulation of the blood. The authors do not include much information about specific drugs and their doses deliberately as this differs in certain countries and settings. Instead we recommend that the reader is familiar with their own local policies and procedures for the pharmacological management of patients.

## Atherosclerosis

Is a process where arteries become hardened by plaques made up of fatty substances, such as cholesterol and triglycerides. The hardening and narrowing of the arteries can reduce the flow of blood and oxygen to the heart muscle causing coronary heart disease. In other arteries the process can cause stroke or peripheral arterial disease.

If a plaque ruptures (Fig. 7.3) it can lead to the formation of a blood clot, known as a thrombus. This clot can then block subsequent blood flow to portions of the heart supplied by the blocked artery (Fig. 7.4). An enzyme named thrombin causes fibrin to be formed from fibrinogen (Fig. 7.5). This mesh of fibrin traps blood cells and platelets. Platelet aggregation is triggered by the damage to the vessels endothelium caused by the rupture. The platelets attach to the exposed collagen by binding to von Willebrand's factors.

The risk factors for coronary heart disease can be split into modifiable and nonmodifiable risk factors (Table 7.3). Modifiable risk factors include things that can be changed or better managed by patients, usually by making certain lifestyle changes. Nonmodifiable risk however are beyond the control or influence of the patient, such as gender and genetic makeup.

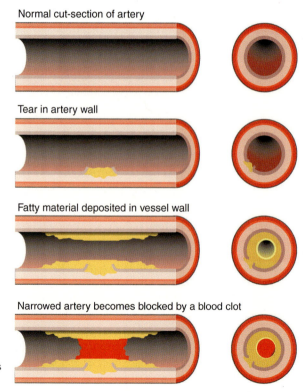

Normal cut-section of artery

Tear in artery wall

Fatty material deposited in vessel wall

Narrowed artery becomes blocked by a blood clot

**Fig. 7.3** Atherosclerosis leading to coronary thrombus formation

**Fig. 7.4** The occlusion in the right coronary artery can be clearly seen. This patient had a collateral vessel allowing blood to bypass the blockage naturally

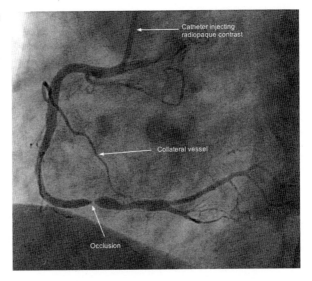

**Fig. 7.5** Thrombus formation leading to myocardial infarction

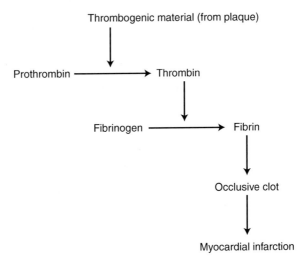

# Angina

The extent of the arterial occlusion can cause symptoms of angina or other acute coronary syndromes. Nitrates, such as; glyceryl trinitrate (GTN), isosorbide mono-nitrate (ISMN) and isosorbide dinitrate (ISDN) are often used to relieve symptoms of angina. Nitrates work by dilating the coronary arteries and increasing blood/ oxygen flow to the heart, whilst simultaneously reducing preload by dilating the systemic veins. Due to the mechanism of action and side effects of nitrates, patients

**Table 7.3**  Modifiable and nonmodifiable coronary heart disease risk factors

| Nonmodifiable | Modifiable |
| --- | --- |
| Age | Smoking |
| Race | High blood cholesterol |
| Sex | High blood pressure |
| Genetics | Obesity and inactivity |
| | Diabetes |

**Fig. 7.6**  Stable angina pectoris

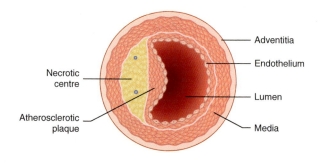

can develop tachycardia, feel dizzy, have headaches and develop postural hypotension. There are several different types of angina, including:

- Stable angina
- Unstable angina
- Prinzmetal's/variant angina

## Stable Angina

Stable angina pectoris (Fig. 7.6) is caused by atherosclerotic plaque(s) in one or more of the coronary arteries reducing blood flow to the heart. The reduced blood flow is not normally noticed during routine activities; but during situations requiring increased myocardial demand, angina symptoms become apparent. Pain is often felt in the chest, neck, jaw or arms and is essentially caused by demand for blood and oxygen being greater than supply. Exercise and emotional stress can trigger an angina attack.

## Unstable Angina

Unlike stable angina, symptoms can also occur during rest. There is significant narrowing of the arterial lumen substantially reducing coronary blood flow (Fig. 7.7).

## Prinzmetal's Angina

Also known as vasospastic or variant angina is a form of angina that is not caused by narrowing of the vessel due to plaques but instead by contraction of the smooth

**Fig. 7.7** Unstable angina pectoris

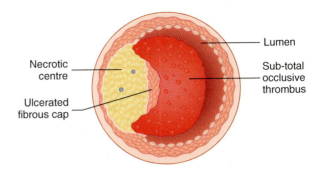

Necrotic centre

Ulcerated fibrous cap

Lumen

Sub-total occlusive thrombus

**Fig. 7.8** Prinzmetal's angina

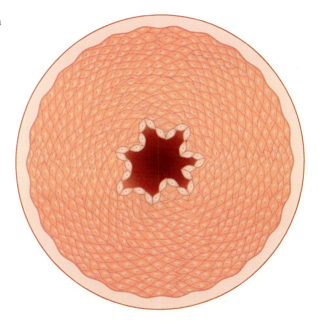

muscle tissue in the vessel termed vasospasm (Fig. 7.8). The narrowing of the artery due to contraction has the effect of reducing the amount of blood and oxygen to the heart leading to angina symptoms. The symptoms can occur at rest and usually at night. Prinzmetal's angina is often seen as transient ST elevation on the ECG, sometimes with hyperacute T waves or T wave inversion. This can make it difficult to identify, as the ECG needs to be performed during an attack to see this effect.

Clues to the presence of angina are seen as ischemic changes on the ECG. These signs of ischemia affect the T wave and ST segment causing either flattening or depression of the T wave/ST segment or the inversion of T waves (Table 7.4 and Fig. 7.9). In addition there are several different appearances to the presentation of ST depression, including upsloping, downsloping and horizontal (Fig. 7.10), which describe the position of the ST segment relative to the isoelectric baseline.

**Table 7.4** Various signs of ischemia on the ECG

| T wave inversion | ST depression | Flattened T wave |
| --- | --- | --- |
| 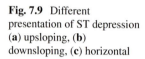 | Isoelectric baseline / ST depression | |

**Fig. 7.9** Different presentation of ST depression (**a**) upsloping, (**b**) downsloping, (**c**) horizontal

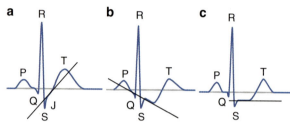

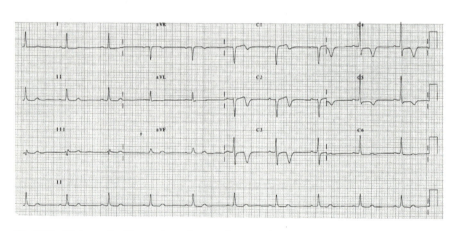

**Fig. 7.10** ST depression/T wave inversion seen in precordial leads

## Digitalis Effect

Another situation which presents with widespread ST depression is digitalis/digoxin effect in which the morphology of the ST depression resembles a tick that is the wrong way around (reverse tick) or a gradual sloping (Figs. 7.11 and 7.12). Digitalis effect is caused by the drug digoxin. The presence of this effect does not imply

**Fig. 7.11** The digoxin effect

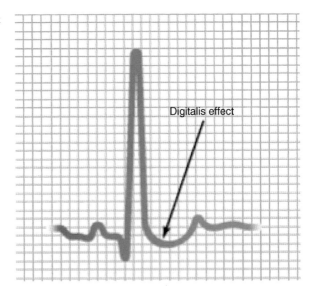

Digitalis effect

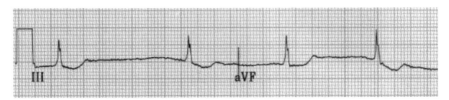

III                    aVF

**Fig. 7.12** The digoxin effect showing clearly the 'reversed tick' ST depression

digoxin toxicity. Further clues to this effect also include a shortened QT interval and possible PR interval prolongation and prominent U waves. A patient drug history is essential to confirm digitalis effect.

## Myocardial Infarction

A myocardial infarction, commonly referred to as a heart attack is a term used to describe injury to the heart muscle caused by a lack of sufficient blood, oxygen and other nutrients (Fig. 7.13). There are two different classifications of myocardial infarction:

- ST elevation myocardial infarction (STEMI)
- Non ST elevation myocardial infarction (NSTEMI)

A myocardial infarction includes a variety of symptoms (Table 7.5) and can present in atypical ways. The most generally recognizable symptoms include a severe and persistent pain in the chest, often described as a crushing, squeezing or burning

**Fig. 7.13** Myocardial
infarction

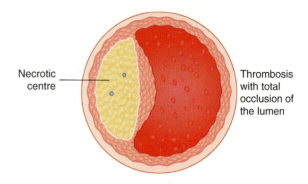

Necrotic
centre

Thrombosis
with total
occlusion of
the lumen

**Table 7.5** Signs and
symptoms of myocardial
infarction

| Chest pain (unrelieved by rest or angina medication) |
| --- |
| Retrosternal location |
| Crushing |
| Squeezing |
| Burning |
| Feeling of impending doom |
| Nausea/vomiting |
| Hypertension or hypotension |
| Shortness of breath |
| Cyanosis |
| Dizziness/collapse |
| Atypical signs and symptoms include: |
| Abdominal pain |
| Pain in the back |
| Pain in the shoulder |
| Pain in the jaw |

pain. The pain often spreads to the neck, arms and/or jaw. Nausea/vomiting, short-
ness of breath and a cold clammy appearance are also frequently observed.
Sometimes patients can present with atypical signs and symptoms, this is more
likely with the elderly and women. Angina pain is usually relieved by rest and
angina medication. If the pain is different to the patients 'normal' angina pain and
persists after rest/medication then myocardial infarction is highly likely.

## *Door to Needle or Balloon Time*

Prompt intervention is vital in cases of suspected MI. The more time goes by, the
more heart muscle is damaged. "Time is muscle" is a phrase often used in cardiology.
The delay to reperfusion of a patient is measured and referred to often as "door to balloon" or "door to needle" time depending on the treatment used (angioplasty or
thrombolysis). Several methods have been introduced in centres around the world to

**Fig. 7.14** ST elevation

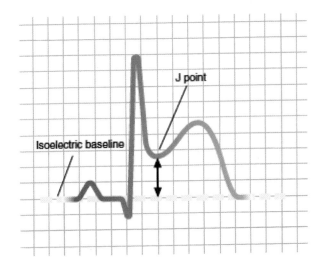

**Table 7.6** Causes of ST segment elevation

| |
|---|
| Acute myocardial infarction |
| Acute pericarditis |
| Acute myocarditis |
| High take off |
| Brugada syndrome |
| Left ventricular aneurysm |
| Prinzmetal's/variant angina |
| Normal variant |
| Intracranial hemorrhage |

reduce these delays for better outcomes. Some include the electronic transmission of prehospital ECGs to specialist units or personnel in hospital, i.e. CCU or a cardiology consultant. Suspected MI patients can then bypass the emergency department and go straight to cardiac cath lab for treatment. Where the nearest cath lab is very far from a patient (i.e. patients living in rural areas) specially trained paramedics have been used to interpret the ECG and inject powerful drugs to break down the thrombus, called thrombolysis. More about these treatment methods is discussed later in the chapter.

## ST Elevation

Before discussing ST elevation myocardial infarctions it is necessary to understand ST elevation. ST elevation refers to the ST segment of the waveform being elevated above the isoelectric baseline (Fig. 7.14).

Elevation is measured in mm from the baseline to the J point. The J point is the junction between the end of the QRS complex and the start of the ST segment. Every lead should be examined in turn for the presence of any ST elevation. There are many conditions that can cause ST elevation (Table 7.6) however ST elevation associated with

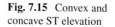
**Fig. 7.15** Convex and concave ST elevation

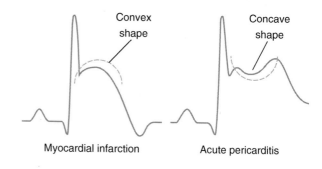

Myocardial infarction                    Acute pericarditis

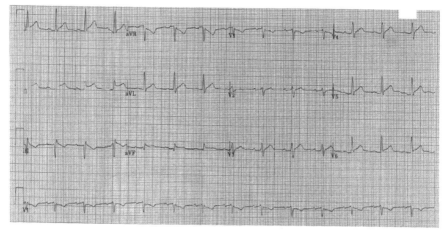

**Fig. 7.16** Pericarditis

myocardial infarction tends to occur in certain leads depending on which coronary arteries are blocked. The ST elevation tends to be convex in shape as oppose to concave, which is seen in other conditions, such as acute pericarditis (Figs. 7.15 and 7.16) where concave ST elevation is present in multiple leads with no reciprocal changes.

High take off or early repolarisation are displayed as ST elevation on the ECG, usually in anterior leads. This can be a normal variant, especially in young black males.

## *J Waves*

J waves or Osborn waves as they are sometimes referred are waves that are located at the junction of the QRS complex and the T wave (Fig. 7.17). They are usually more symmetrical in appearance and often look like a second smaller QRS complex. They are present in conditions such as hypothermia, hypercalcaemia, head injuries and sometimes a normal finding in some patients. J waves can sometimes be confused with ST elevation.

**Fig. 7.17** A J wave

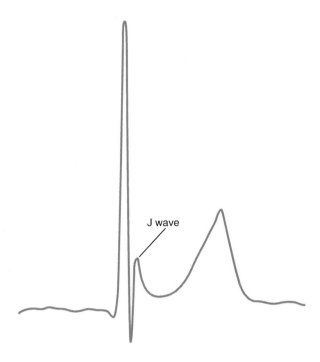

J wave

## *STEMI*

A STEMI is a type of myocardial infarction that is characterised by ST elevation on the ECG in certain lead areas termed territories. Sometimes a STEMI may also be referred to as a Q wave infarction. The blockage prevents blood, oxygen and other nutrients reaching the heart muscle past the occlusion. This leads to muscle death and akinesia (lack of movement in that part of the heart muscle).

ST elevation indicates myocardial injury as the injured area or zone that surrounds the zone of infarction remains electrically positive, leading to ST elevation (Fig. 7.18).

In addition to the ST segment elevation, the presence of pathological Q waves is a key feature of an STEMI. Pathological Q waves are >0.03 s or 30 ms in width and a quarter the height of the R wave. Q waves are seen because of myocardial necrosis occurring in the zone of infarction. ECG leads in proximity to the infarction only detect electrical impulses in the right ventricle and septum moving away from the lead. This occurs because the necrosed tissue is electrically inert. Pathological Q waves usually develop between 12 and 24 hours after the start of a myocardial infarction. Table 7.7 summarises the morphological changes seen on the ECG to waveforms affected by the zones of ischemia, injury and infarction.

**Fig. 7.18** Myocardial
infarction

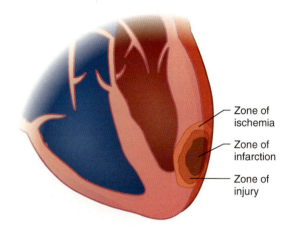

Zone of
ischemia

Zone of
infarction

Zone of
injury

**Table 7.7** Morphological changes to the ECG waveform from ischemia to necrosis

| Ischemia | Injury | Infarction |
|---|---|---|
| T wave and/or ST segment changes caused by altered repolarisation | ST elevation indicates myocardial injury | Pathological Q waves idicating infarction and necrosis of cardiac tissue |

**Evolution of a STEMI**

Several key changes occur to the waveform over time during a STEMI (Fig. 7.19).
Minutes to hours after the start of a MI, elevation of the ST segment or hyperacute
T waves may be seen. Within hours to a day the formation of large pathological Q
waves occurs with T wave inversion. Over weeks to months the ST segment and T
wave normalise with the exception of the Q wave. Sometimes the T wave also
remains inverted. Old myocardial infarctions are often identifiable by the presence
of Q waves in the territory of the previous MI.

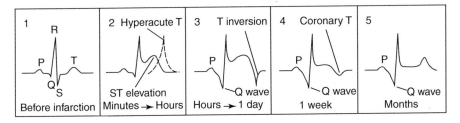

| 1<br>R | 2 Hyperacute T | 3   T inversion | 4   Coronary T | 5 |
|---|---|---|---|---|
| P       T<br>Q<br> S | ST elevation | P<br>~Q wave | P<br>~Q wave | P<br>~Q wave |
| Before infarction | Minutes → Hours | Hours → 1 day | 1 week | Months |

**Fig. 7.19**  Evolution of a STEMI

**Fig. 7.20**  Tombstoning

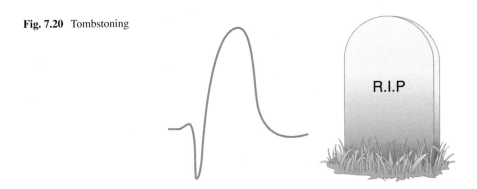

## Ventricular Aneurysm

A complication that may arise following a myocardial infarction is a ventricular aneurysm. This is seen in the case of left ventricular aneurysms on the ECG as persistent ST elevation and the presence of Q waves visible months after the MI. These aneurysms are caused by weakened areas of the ventricular wall expanding with blood which may lead to subsequent reduction of blood flow.

## Tombstoning

Is term often used to describe ST elevation where the J point and T wave are elevated resembling a tombstone (Fig. 7.20). Tombstoning has been associated with a poorer prognosis; also a greater percentage of patients exhibiting tombstoning go on to develop life threatening arrhythmias.

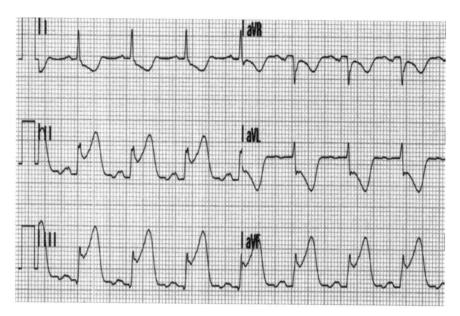

**Fig. 7.21**  Reciprocal changes seen clearly in the anterior leads I and aVL

## Reciprocal Changes

This refers to a phenomenon where the changes made to the damaged region of the heart by injury, infarction or ischemia are seen in mirror image in opposite leads. This means that positive changes are mirrored negatively. An example of this can be seen in Fig. 7.21, which shows an ECG with clear ST elevation in the inferior leads (II, III and aVF). Reciprocal changes can be seen in the anterior leads (I and aVL). The presence of reciprocal changes adds additional evidence to support the presence of an acute myocardial infarction. The mechanism causing these changes is not yet understood however patients presenting with reciprocal changes have a higher mortality rate than those with ST elevation alone.

## MI Regions/Territories

The location of the ST elevation on the ECG can give a clue as to which vessel or vessels are affected (Fig. 7.22 and Table 7.8).

Knowing the territory of the MI and the level of ST elevation gives clues as to the potential severity of the occlusion. There can be combination of territories involved. For example ST elevation may be seen in both the inferior and lateral leads, or the anterior and lateral leads making the MI an inferolateral or anterolateral STEMI respectively. Figure 7.23 shows an example of an inferior MI with extensive ST

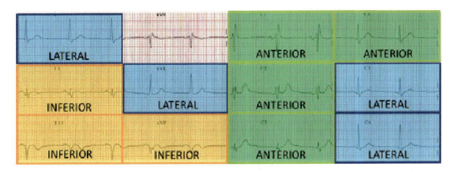

**Fig. 7.22** MI regions

**Table 7.8** MI regions (NB: the artery may not always correspond to the leads due to anatomical variance)

| Leads | Reciprocal leads | Colour codes | Area of the heart | Probable artery involved |
|---|---|---|---|---|
| II, III, aVF | I, aVL | Orange | Inferior | Right coronary artery |
| I, aVL, $V_5$, $V_6$ | II, III, aVF | Blue | Lateral | Circumflex artery |
| $V_1$, $V_2$, $V_3$, $V_4$ | None | Green | Anterior | Left anterior descending<br><br>NB: Leads $V_1$ and $V_2$ represent septal regions |

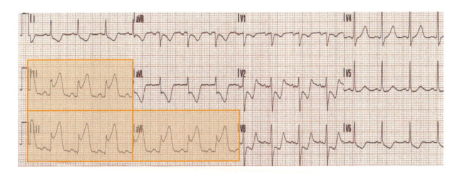

**Fig. 7.23** Inferior STEMI

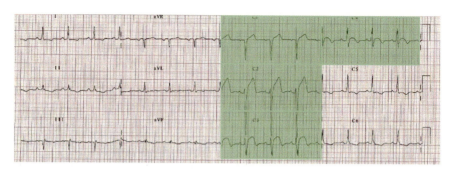

**Fig. 7.24** Anterior STEMI

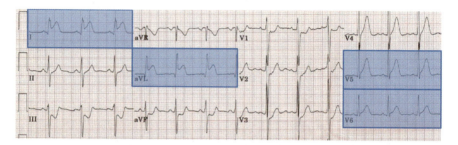

**Fig. 7.25** Lateral STEMI [Life in the Fast Lane (http://lifeinthefastlane.com/education/procedures/lead-positioning/)/CC BY-SA 4.0 (http://creativecommons.org/licenses/by-sa/4.0/)]

elevation in the inferior leads II, III and aVF. The pattern of ST depression in leads $V_2$ and $V_3$ also suggests the presence of a coexisting posterior MI making the ECG an inferior-posterior STEMI. Examples of anterior and lateral STEMI can be seen in Figs. 7.24 and 7.25.

## Posterior and Right Ventricular MI

Recording a posterior ECG may also be of benefit if a posterior MI is suspected. Posterior MI's usually occur in the presence of lateral or inferior MI's but can also occur in isolation. They are suspected when certain changes occur in the leads $V_1$, $V_2$ and $V_3$, including; positively deflected T waves, ST depression and dominant tall/broad R waves (Fig. 7.26). If you were to turn the ECG upside down it would resemble a STEMI in the leads showing the posterior changes (Fig. 7.27).

To better view a suspected posterior MI, a posterior ECG is recorded. This is done by relocating the chest leads $V_4$, $V_5$ and $V_6$ to the patients back (on the left side) as seen in Fig. 7.28. They are then referred to respectively as $V_7$, $V_8$ and $V_9$. When the ECG is printed the practitioner should relabel the leads accordingly to

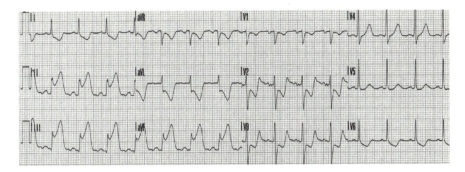

**Fig. 7.26** Inferior-posterior STEMI

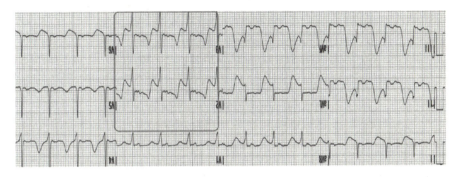

**Fig. 7.27** The same ECG (Fig. 7.26) upside down

**Fig. 7.28** Posterior lead placement

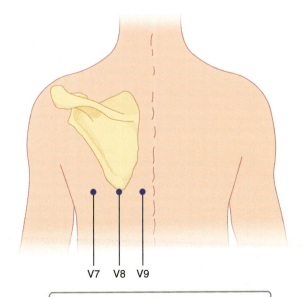

$V_7$ - Left posterior axillary line, in line with $V_4$
$V_8$ - Below the posterior tip of the scapula, in line with $V_4$
$V_9$ - The edge of the spine, in line with $V_4$

**Table 7.9** Relabeling of chest leads for a posterior lead recording

| $V_4$ | $V_7$ |
|---|---|
| $V_5$ | $V_8$ |
| $V_6$ | $V_9$ |

**Fig. 7.29** Right sided chest lead placement

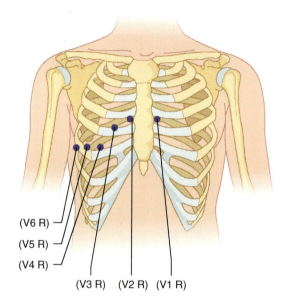

(V6 R)
(V5 R)
(V4 R)
(V3 R)   (V2 R)   (V1 R)

**Table 7.10** Additional reasons for right sided ECG recording

| Note: There are other indications for recording a right sided ECG, including: |
|---|
| In young children with a dominant right ventricle |
| People with dextrocardia |
| Right ventricular infarction |

show that the ECG was recorded with posterior leads (Table 7.9). Posterior MIs can then be confirmed by the presence of ST elevation and Q waves in leads $V_7$–$V_9$.

Infarction of the right ventricle occurs in just under half the cases of inferior MI but will not be seen on the ECG. One way to detect them is to record a right sided ECG (Fig. 7.29) this basically works by applying the chest leads in the normal positions but on the right side of the chest instead of the left. The letter 'R' should also written next to each lead on the ECG to indicate that this is a right sided lead. For speed practitioners sometimes just move the $V_4$ lead and place it on the right side of the chest and label it $V_4$R on the ECG after a standard recording to view the right ventricle. Right sided ECGs are also recorded for several other reasons apart from right ventricular infarction, as highlighted in Table 7.10.

**Table 7.11** Biomarkers type and peak action

| Marker | Type | Peak action (h) |
|---|---|---|
| Troponin T and Troponin I | Regulatory proteins | >12 |
| Creatine Kinase (CK) | Enzyme | >24 |
| Aspartate aminotransferase (AST) | Non-specific enzyme | >30 |
| Lactate dehydrogenase (LDH) | Non-specific enzyme | >48 |

## LBBB and Chest Pain

A LBBB can make it very difficult to spot signs of ischemia and/or ST elevation. Therefore any patient presenting with a new LBBB and chest pain or other symptoms of ACS should be treated as a medical emergency and receive further investigations to identify the underlying cause.

Sgarbossa's criteria is a point based system to help identify the possibility of a STEMI in patients with a LBBB. This is discussed in more detail in Chap. 5.

## NSTEMI

Or non ST elevation MI is a form of myocardial infarction where ST elevation is not evidenced on the ECG. NSTEMI's are sometimes referred to as non Q wave MIs. Although still a medical emergency they are usually less serious than STEMIs, as a smaller section of the heart is damaged due to the clot only partially occluding the artery.

To help distinguish between unstable angina and a NSTEMI, bloods are taken to look for changes in cardiac biomarkers that are indicative of myocardial damage. These changes may not be detectable for up to 12 h or more. Another clue is that the ST/T waves changes are usually transient in unstable angina but tend to persist with NSTEMI.

## Cardiac Biomarkers

Can be measured to give an indication of damage to the heart. Necrosis of myocardial cells can be seen by examining troponins, which are specific and sensitive markers. Other markers are also measured, including; troponin T, troponin I, creatine kinase (CK/CK-MB), lactate dehydrogenase (LDH) and aspartate aminotransaminase (AST). These biomarkers reach their peak serum volumes at different times. The troponins are the quickest to peak at 12 h. Troponin is often measured on admission and 12 h later when a patient is admitted with a suspected NSTEMI. The level usually normalises at 48 h. The commonly measured biomarkers and their peak action time can be seen in Table 7.11.

**Table 7.12**  other causes of
raised troponin levels

| Sepsis |
| --- |
| Renal failure |
| Defibrillation |
| Post heart transplant |
| Pulmonary embolism |
| Pericarditis |
| Myocarditis |
| Heart failure |
| Atrial fibrillation |

**Fig. 7.30**  Thrombolytic
action

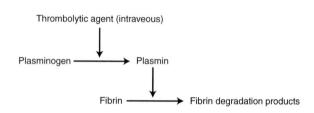

It is also important to be aware that many other conditions can cause elevation of
Troponin levels (Table 7.12). The patients biomarkers, ECG and history of the presenting complaint should all be taken into account before assuming an acute coronary syndrome is present.

## Treatment for Myocardial Infarction

Myocardial infarction can be treated in several ways, including pharmacologically,
using powerful clot busting drugs referred to as thrombolytic therapy. Patients may
also be treated by angioplasty in a cardiac cath lab where balloons and stents are
used to open the blocked vessels. These interventions are discussed in more detail
below.

**Thrombolytic Therapy**

Thrombolytics are a group of drugs that act to break down thrombi. For example
Streptokinase is a fibrinolytic agent that acts on plasminogen to produce a fibrinolytic enzyme called plasmin which breaks down clots (Fig. 7.30). Some of the commonly used thrombolytic drugs are listed in Table 7.13.

There are several risks associated with the use of thrombolytic therapy, where
contraindications (Table 7.14) are not present then these risks are relatively low
compared to the potential benefits. The risk of stroke for instance is less than
1 % whereas there is a 50 % reduction in the risk of death from acute myocardial

| **Table 7.13** Commonly used thrombolytic drugs | Streptokinase |
|---|---|
| | Alteplase |
| | Tenecteplase |
| | Reteplase |

| **Table 7.14** Contraindications for thrombolysis | A normal ECG |
|---|---|
| | History of stroke or known intracranial pathology |
| | Bleeding disorder |
| | Uncontrolled hypertension |
| | Current GI bleeding |
| | Previous administration of streptokinase (if using streptokinase again) |
| | Recent surgery or trauma |

infarction when thrombolytic therapy is used. For this therapy to be used patients must not have any absolute contraindications and posses ST elevation of ≥1 mm in two adjacent limb leads or ≥2 mm in two adjacent precordial leads. Chest pain with a new left bundle branch block is also criteria for eligibility.

Percutaneous coronary intervention or PCI also known as angioplasty is a process carried out in a cardiac catheterisation lab where catheters are placed into the coronary arteries allowing radio opaque contrast to be injected so the arteries can be viewed by x-ray. This allows for visualisation of the coronary arteries. Small balloons can then be inflated to squash the blockage and restore blood flow to the artery. Small metal cages called stents (Figs. 7.31 and 7.32) can also placed to keep the artery open.

Coronary artery bypass grafts (CABG) may also be used to treat atherosclerosis or when a PCI fails. If there are widespread blockages in multiple vessels, coronary artery bypass grafts may be a more suitable treatment. Bypass grafts are made by attaching veins, arteries or both to the aorta or left subclavian artery and then attaching them to a blocked coronary artery after the point of blockage acting to bypass the blockage (Fig. 7.33). Arterial grafts have a longer life than venous grafts with a patency rate of >70 % at 10 years in some cases. The long or short saphenous vein, radial artery and left internal mammary artery are frequently used to bypass blocked arteries. It is also possible to carry out angioplasty to subsequently blocked bypass grafts.

There are various pros and cons to angioplasty and CABG. Angioplasty requires a shorter hospital stay, faster return to work and lower mortality risk than CABG. However a significant number of patients receiving angioplasty may require further treatment within 6 months of the procedure. Although risk and recovery time are higher in CABG patients they tend to have less need for further surgery or angioplasty within a year.

**Fig. 7.31** Percutaneous
coronary intervention (PCI)

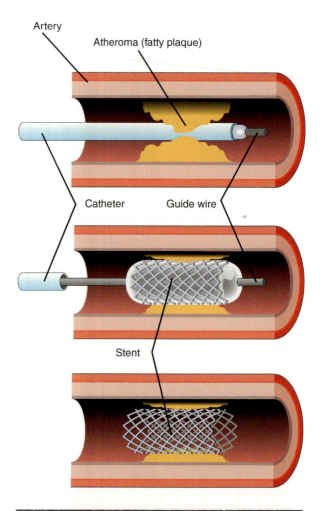

Artery

Atheroma (fatty plaque)

Catheter                    Guide wire

Stent

**Fig. 7.32** A photograph of a
stent

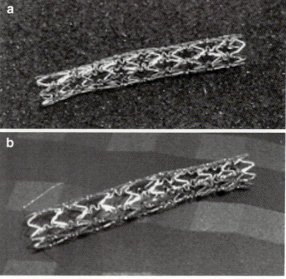

**Fig. 7.33** Coronary artery bypass grafts

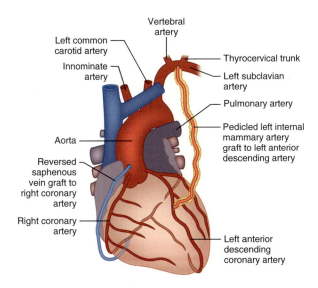

Vertebral artery

Left common carotid artery

Innominate artery

Thyrocervical trunk

Left subclavian artery

Pulmonary artery

Aorta

Pedicled left internal mammary artery graft to left anterior descending artery

Reversed saphenous vein graft to right coronary artery

Right coronary artery

Left anterior descending coronary artery

Some patients are not suitable for either bypass surgery or angioplasty. These patients may be managed medically or in some cases offered laser treatment to destroy nerve fibres, preventing angina pain. There is also a theory that the laser treatment may stimulate angiogenesis. The procedure is referred to as transmyocardial revascularization.

### The Intra Aortic Balloon Pump (IABP)

This is a device used to increase oxygen supply to the myocardium and cardiac output improving the coronary artery blood flow by means of counterpulsation. A catheter with a large balloon is passed percutaneously into the femoral artery and placed below the aortic arch using fluoroscopic imaging. The inflation and deflation of the balloon is timed to occur during diastole and systole to provide circulatory support to the patient (Fig. 7.34, Table 7.15).

### Reperfusion Arrhythmias

Some patients develop a reperfusion arrhythmia following restoration of blood flow. There are two frequently seen types. Idioventricular and accelerated idioventricular rhythm. The most common of which is accelerated Idioventricular rhythm.

Idioventricular rhythm is essentially an escape rhythm where the dominant pacemaker originates from lower down in the ventricles preventing asystole. It appears on the ECG with wide QRS complexes a rate between 20 and 40 BPM (Fig. 7.35).

Accelerated idioventricular rhythm is sometimes referred to as slow VT and has a rate of between 40 and 120 BPM. The rhythm is considered benign and does not usually require treatment.

**Fig. 7.34** Action of the
IABP

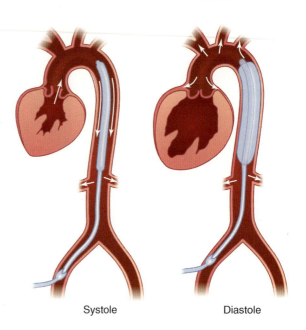

Systole                     Diastole

**Table 7.15** Balloon action
associated with myocardial
contraction

| Diastole | Systole |
|----------|---------|
| Inflation of balloon | Deflation of balloon |

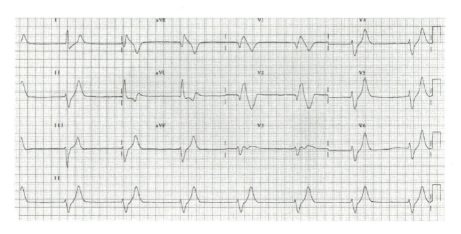

**Fig. 7.35** Idioventricular rhythm

## Summary of Key Points

- Acute coronary syndromes are medical emergencies requiring prompt intervention.
- Acute coronary syndromes comprise of unstable angina, STEMI and NSTEMI.
- Atherosclerosis is the main cause of narrowing and subsequent coronary artery blockages
- The presence of ST elevation in certain lead territories combined with the presence of reciprocal changes is highly suggestive of ST elevation myocardial infarction
- The diagnosis between unstable angina and NSTEMI is based on the results of cardiac biomarkers detected in blood
- Acute myocardial infarction sometimes presents in atypical ways, particularly with women and the elderly
- Time is critical to the treatment of myocardial infarction, the more time passes the more extensive the myocardial damage

## Quiz

Q1. The presence of widespread ST depression resembling a reverse tick may indicate.
   (A) Parkinsons disease
   (B) Digoxin/digitalis effect
   (C) STEMI

Q2. Which of the following lead combinations are known as the inferior leads?
   (A) I, aVL, $V_5$ and $V_6$
   (B) $V_1$, $V_2$, $V_3$ and $V_4$
   (C) II, III and aVF

Q3. Persistent ST elevation with pathological Q waves lasting longer than 3 months could be a sign of.
   (A) Left ventricular aneurysm
   (B) Left ventricular hypertrophy
   (C) Atrial bigeminy

Q4. One of the reasons a practitioner may record a right sided ECG could be.
   (A) Right handed patients
   (B) Anyone with an intracranial bleed
   (C) On a patient with dextrocardia

Q5. Prinzmetal's angina is caused by.
   (A) Atherosclerosis
   (B) Vasospasm
   (C) Thrombolysis

Q6. An example of a platelet aggregation inhibitor would be.

   (A)  Aspirin
   (B)  Warfarin
   (C)  Ramipril

Interpret the following ECGs

**Q7.**

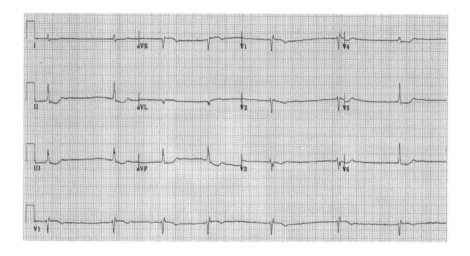

**Q8.**

**Q9.**

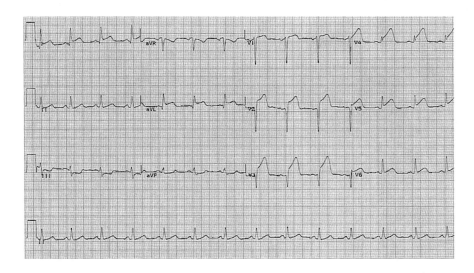

Answers: Q1 = B, Q2 = C, Q3 = A, Q4 = C, Q5 = B, Q6 = A, Q7 = digoxin effect, Q8 = pericarditis, Q9 = anterolateral STEMI

# Chapter 8
# Genetic Cardiac Conditions

**Keywords** Genetics • Genes • Brugada • Mutation • Chromosomes • Autosomal • Dominant • Recessive

## Background

There are many genetically acquired cardiac diseases. To understand the pathology of this group of diseases, a basic knowledge of genetics is required.

Eukaryotic cells contain a nucleus, which stores chromosomes, which in turn contains DNA (deoxyribonucleic acid) (Fig. 8.1). DNA consists of sections called genes that determine various physical traits.

Germline cells, such as the gametes, which include sperm and ova cells allow genetic material to be passed onto children; as oppose to the somatic cells (all the other cells in the body) whose genetic material is not passed on to children. Each gamete consists of 23 chromosomes, which when combined, make the full complement of 46 chromosomes that most humans posses.

Mutations in genes can lead to various diseases. These mutations can be passed on to children from their parents. If a gene allele has a particular dominant trait it gains precedence over less dominant traits (Fig. 8.2). For example in autosomal dominant inheritance only one of the parents needs to have the mutated gene for it to be passed onto the children. Each child would have a 50 % chance of inheriting the condition. In contrast autosomal recessive inheritance requires both parents to have the genetic defect. This would mean that a child would have a 25 % chance of developing the disease and 50 % chance of inheriting an abnormal gene, which would make the child a carrier of the disease. It is also possible for a new gene mutation to occur in the gametes, termed a 'de novo' mutation. In this case the child develops the condition without either parent having the disease, or being a carrier.

It is worth noting that there are many other patterns of genetic inheritance, which are beyond the scope of this book (Table 8.1).

© Springer-Verlag London 2015
A. Davies, A. Scott, *Starting to Read ECGs: A Comprehensive Guide to Theory and Practice*, DOI 10.1007/978-1-4471-4965-1_8

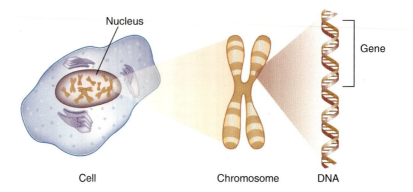

**Fig. 8.1** Location of genes within a cell

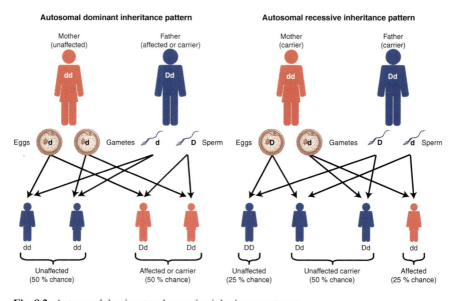

**Fig. 8.2** Autosomal dominant and recessive inheritance patterns

**Table 8.1** Other inheritance patterns

| |
| --- |
| Autosomal dominant |
| Autosomal recessive |
| X-linked dominant |
| X-linked recessive |
| Mitochondrial |
| Co-dominant |

# Brugada Syndrome

Brugada syndrome is a condition that is associated with a significant increase in the risk of sudden death in young adults and sometimes children. The condition was first accepted as a clinical condition in 1992 based on the work of Pedro and Josep Brugada. Brugada syndrome affects males more than females. Disease prevalence is estimated at 1–5 per 10,000 people and has a high frequency of occurrence in Southeast Asia, especially in Thailand and the Philippines. In contrast there is a lower frequency of cases in western countries.

Brugada has been linked with a mutation in the SCN5A (Fig. 8.3) gene that encodes the α-subunit of the human cardiac sodium channel. Coding is a set of rules that are applied to DNA or mRNA (messenger ribonucleic acid) that translates them into proteins, which in turn consist of chains of amino acids. A mutation in this process can lead to variations that can cause certain positive effects, such as increased resistance to a disease for example; or negative effects, as seen in conditions like cystic fibrosis and Brugada syndrome.

Apart from SCN5A, which accounts for around 20 % of cases of Brugada syndrome, several other calcium-channel mutations have been identified i.e. CACNB2, CACNA1C, SCN1B and GDP1L.

The mutation that occurs in brugada leads to ion channel defects, which either: Reduce the sodium or calcium influx into the cell or increase potassium efflux from the cell.

Brugada is an autosomal dominant disease. This means that the abnormal gene can be inherited if only one parent has the condition rather than both. This means that children of a parent with Brugada syndrome have a 50 % chance of inheriting the condition. It is also possible for a spontaneous mutation in either of the parents gametes (sperm or ova) to result in a de novo mutation (a new mutation not seen in either parent) causing Brugada syndrome.

Brugada syndrome is characterised by a Right Bundle Branch Block (RBBB) pattern with persistent ST-elevation in the precordial leads ($V_1$–$V_3$). The ECG is

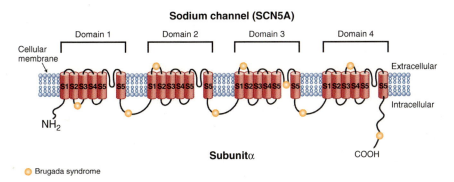

**Fig. 8.3** Effects of Brugada syndrome on the sodium channel

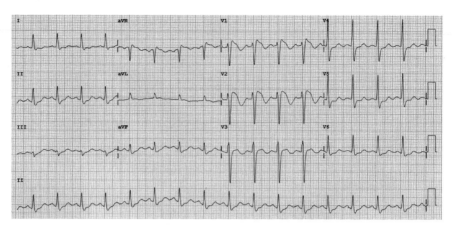

**Fig. 8.4** Brugada syndrome (type 1)

| **Table 8.2** Other causes of the Brugada ECG pattern | |
|---|---|
| | Abnormal right bundle branch block (RBBB) |
| | Acute myocardial infarction (MI) or pericarditis |
| | Pulmonary embolism (PE) |
| | Hyperkalemia |
| | Hypercalcemia |
| | Hypothermia |
| | Early repolarization |
| | Left ventricular hypertrophy (LVH) |
| | Arrhythmogenic right ventricular dysplasia (ARVD) |
| | Cardiomyopathy |
| | Duchenne muscular dystrophy (DMD) |

often very dynamic and frequently masks the presence of the syndrome. Brugada can however be revealed by certain physical states, such as hyperthermia and some drugs, for example sodium-channel blockers. Other signs can include a low heart rate at night, which may predispose patients in the group to an increased risk of Ventricular Fibrillation (VF). Brugada patients are also at an increased risk of developing Atrial Fibrillation (AF), which is seen in around 20 % of Brugada syndrome patients. Syncope or Sudden Cardiac Death (SCD) can also be the first clinical manifestation of the condition. Figure 8.4 shows an example of Brugada syndrome.

There are three main types of Brugada syndrome, types 1–3. Type 1 is characterised by coved ST-elevation with a negatively deflected T-wave. Type 2 differs in that the ST-elevation is saddle back in appearance and the T-wave is often biphasic or positively deflected. Finally type 3 can have the coved or saddleback appearance of the earlier types but with less ST-elevation (<1 mm). When considering Brugada it is also worth eliminating other causes of the Brugada ECG pattern (Table 8.2).

Genetic testing is recommended in addition to clinical findings to support the diagnosis and to detect relatives at risk of developing the condition so they can receive appropriate counselling and treatment if appropriate.

> **Note**
> Moving the chest leads on the right up to the second or third intercostal spaces may increase the chances of detecting the abnormalities associated with Brugada syndrome

## *Treatment*

Although Quinidine (a class I antiarrhythmic agent) has shown some promise in clinical trials, the gold standard for both secondary prevention for those with Brugada syndrome, and for survivors of a cardiac arrest with Brugada syndrome, is an implantable cardiac defibrillator (Table 8.3). The use of sodium-channel blockers (e.g. flecainide, procainamide, ajmaline, pilsicainide) can be used as a drug challenge to help unmask Brugada syndrome. Other drugs that can also reveal the syndrome are listed in Table 8.4.

**Table 8.3** What is an ICD (implantable cardiac defibrillator)

| 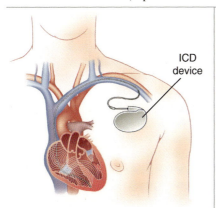 ICD device | An ICD is a medical device implanted in a pocket made in the chest. This device has leads (wires) inside the ventricle. Electrical pulses or shocks can be delivered to the heart to prevent or treat a cardiac arrest |
| --- | --- |

**Table 8.4** Drugs that can reveal the presence of Brugada syndrome

| |
| --- |
| Tricyclic antidepressants |
| Vagotonic agents |
| Beta blockers |
| Intoxication (alcohol/cocaine) |

## Lev's Disease

Lev's disease, also known as Lenegre-Lev syndrome is characterised by fibrosis and calcification of the His-Purkinje system. The disease is a form of idiopathic (no known cause) fibrosis that leads to a form of acquired complete heart block that is usually treated by insertion of a permanent pacemaker. This condition is usually seen in the elderly.

Although the disease was independently described by both Maurice Lev and a frenchman named Jean Lenègre, sometimes Lev's disease is used to refer to fibrosis of the distal His-Purkinje system in the elderly, whereas Lenègre's disease describes fibrosis of the proximal His-Purkinje system in younger patients. Some studies have also shown a link between mutations of SCN5A and the disease.

## Duchenne Muscular Dystrophy

There are several different forms of muscular dystrophy (Table 8.5). Duchenne Muscular Dystrophy (DMD) is a progressive muscle wasting disease caused by mutation of the dystrophin gene (part of the X chromosome). DMD is a hereditary sex-linked (X-linked) recessive disorder that affects boys. Females are typically carriers of the disease. The son of a mother who is a carrier will have a 50 % chance of inheriting the disease, whereas a daughter of the same mother will also have a 50 % chance of becoming a carrier.

**Sex-Determination System**
The male (XY) and female (XX) sex-chromosomes. These chromosomes control the sexual characteristics the person will have. For example development of the sexual organs: penis, testicles or vagina

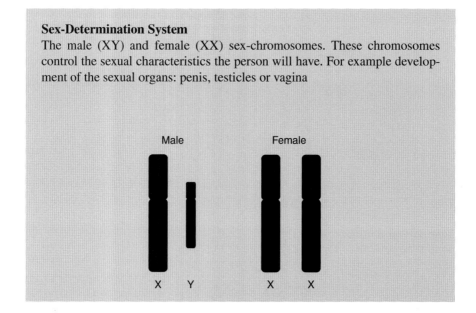

| Table 8.5 Muscular dystrophies | There are various forms of muscular dystrophy that vary in severity and the muscle group(s) affected, they include: |
|---|---|
| | Duchenne |
| | Becker |
| | Emery-Dreifuss |
| | Limb girdle |
| | Facioscapulo-humeral/Landouzy-Dejerine (FSHD) |
| | Oculopharyngeal (OPMD) |

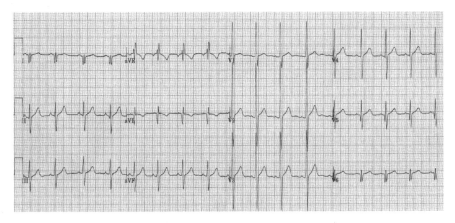

**Fig. 8.5** Muscular dystrophy [Life in the Fast Lane (http://lifeinthefastlane.com/education/proce-dures/lead-positioning/)/CC BY-SA 4.0 (http://creativecommons.org/licenses/by-sa/4.0/)]

Symptoms of the disease usually appear around the ages of 1–3 years. Diagnosis of DMD is usually made through a combination of blood tests (creatine kinase), muscle biopsy and/or genetic tests. There is however a distinct ECG pattern present in DMD that can be a useful indicator to the presence of the disease and to help to distinguish DMD from other forms of muscular dystrophy.

ECG findings in DMD include: Tall R waves in $V_1$, an abnormal R/S ratio in $V_1$ (i.e. RSr pattern), deep Q waves (usually in $V_5$ and $V_6$). Features of incomplete RBBB are often seen (Fig. 8.5). Sinus tachycardia is also often reported. This specific pattern for DMD helps to distinguish Duchenne's from other forms of muscular dystrophy. Thus the ECG in DMD cases can be a useful diagnostic aid.

## Long QT Syndromes

Apart from certain types of drugs, long QT syndrome can also be caused by two genetic conditions: Romano-Ward syndrome and Jervell and Lange-Nielsen syndrome. Both of these syndromes are rare.

## *Romano-Ward Syndrome*

Genetic mutations can affect the function and structure of sodium and potassium ion channels, causing prolongation of the QT interval. Romano-Ward is an autosomal dominant syndrome and is the most common form of genetically acquired long QT syndrome. Several gene mutations have been identified as being linked to the condition, these include: ANK2, KCNE1, KCNE2, KCNQ1 (previously KVLQT1), KCNH2 and SCN5A.

A long QT interval predisposes individuals to ventricular arrhythmias, such as Torsades de pointes and VF. These attacks are often triggered by stimulation of the sympathetic nervous system (i.e. following stress or exercise).

Symptoms can include cardiac arrest, sudden death and episodes of syncope. Paradoxically patients may also experience periods of intermittent bradycardia. Family history can also be important in establishing a diagnosis if there is a history of sudden death or syncope.

### Treatment

An Implantable Cardiac Defibrillator (ICD) is often used, especially in cases of cardiac arrest. Treatment can also include the use of drug therapy (betablockers). If drugs are unsuccessful then surgery can be considered, as it can also be effective in treating some people with long QT syndrome. A procedure called a cervical sympathectomy involves either blocking or completely removing nerves (the left cervical ganglia) from the left side of the neck. This has the effect of reducing the amount of adrenaline that the nerves can deliver to the heart.

## *Jervell and Lange-Nielsen Syndrome*

Less common than Romano-Ward syndrome, Jervell and Lange-Nielsen syndrome is an autosomal recessive condition that is often associated with congenital hearing loss. The vast majority of cases are caused by mutations in the KCNE1 and KCNQ1 genes.

Treatment options are the same as for Romano-Ward with the possible addition of a cochlear implant to help with the hearing loss.

Patients with a Romano-Ward or Jervell and Lange-Nielsen syndrome should avoid any drugs known to prolong the QT interval (Table 8.6).

| **Table 8.6** Drugs that may prolong the QT interval | Some tricyclic antidepressants |
| --- | --- |
| | Some anti-arrhythmogenics |
| | Some antibiotics (e.g. Voriconazole) |

# Arrhythmogenic Right Ventricular Dysplasia/ Cardiomyopathy (ARVD/C)

ARVD/C is an autosomal dominant disease that is marked by various structural changes and arrhythmias that affect the right ventricle. ARVD/C is discussed in more detail with other cardiomyopathies in Chap. 4.

## Summary of Key Points

- There are many genetic conditions that can lead to cardiac problems.
- Many of these conditions can be identified at least in part by ECG changes.
- There are many different mechanisms for inheriting or developing genetic conditions.
- A basic understanding of genetics can aid the practitioner in their understanding of these diseases, and the potential wider implications for patients families, who may also require genetic screening.
- Patients with long-QT syndromes should avoid any drugs that further prolong the QT interval.
- Any patient at risk of sudden cardiac death should have an urgent referral to a cardiologist.

## Quiz

Q1. It is impossible for a child to develop a genetic disease without at least one of the parents having the disease themselves.

   (A) True
   (B) False

Q2. The gold standard treatment for Brugada syndrome is?

   (A) Quinidine
   (B) An Implanted Cardiac Defibrillator (ICD)
   (C) Steroids

Q3. Lev's disease is usually seen in.

   (A) Infants
   (B) The mid to late 20s
   (C) The elderly

Q4. Congenital deafness is associated with.

   (A) Jervell and Lange-Nielsen syndrome
   (B) Romano-Ward syndrome

Q5. Brugada syndrome is more prevalent in.

    (A) The west
    (B) Central Europe
    (C) Southeast Asia

Q6. Tricyclic antidepressants can prolong the QT interval?

    (A) True
    (B) False

Q7. An autosomal dominant inheritance disease pattern means.

    (A) Only one parent needs to be affected or a carrier for the offspring to stand a chance of inheriting the disease.
    (B) Both parents must be affected or carriers.
    (C) Neither parent can be a carrier.

Q8. A cervical sympathectomy (removal of nerves) can be a treatment option for patients with.

    (A) Complete heart block
    (B) Romano-Ward syndrome
    (C) Brugada syndrome

Q9. Identify the following ECG

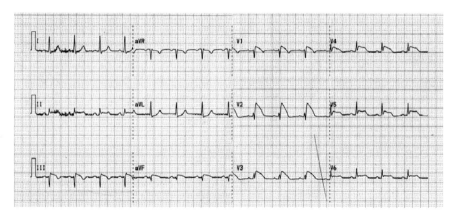

Answers:  Q1=B,  Q2=B,  Q3=C,  Q4=A,  Q5=C,  Q6=A,  Q7=A,  Q8=B, Q9=Brugada syndrome (type 1)

# Chapter 9
# The Pediatric ECG

**Keywords** Pediatric • Children • Infants • Development • Congenital • Defect •
Dextrocardia

## Background

This book focuses primarily on adult conditions. There are many books dedicated
to the interpretation of paediatric ECGs. However the authors believe that it is
appropriate to offer an introduction to the paediatric ECG, as this may benefit
those professionals who work in areas, such as accident and emergency or pre
hospital care that have to regularly deal with patients of all ages. In addition, an
understanding of the development of the heart and the normal values for children
may be of interest to those wishing to deepen their understanding in the field of
cardiology.

## Stages of Myocardial Development

The heart becomes the complex organ we are familiar with from a fairly simple
starting point in the developing embryo. As myocardial development continues the
heart begins to loop taking on an 'S' shape. The septa partition the atria and ventricles from each other and develop simultaneously in the normal heart. Some of the
key stages of development can be seen in Fig. 9.1.

As the heart develops one can acquire various congenital defects that
vary in incidence and severity. Some of the most common are described here
(Table 9.1).

© Springer-Verlag London 2015
A. Davies, A. Scott, *Starting to Read ECGs: A Comprehensive Guide
to Theory and Practice*, DOI 10.1007/978-1-4471-4965-1_9

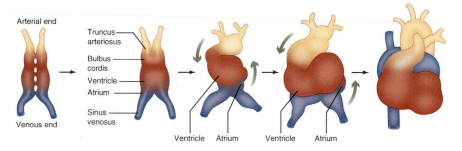

**Fig. 9.1** The stages of cardiac development

**Table 9.1** Summary of commonly encountered congenital heart defects

| Congenital defect | Schematic | Occurrence/births (approx) |
| --- | --- | --- |
| **Coarctation of the aorta** Narrowing of aorta leading to hypertension and left ventricular hypertrophy | Narrowed aorta | 1:1,500 |

**Table 9.1** (continued)

| Congenital defect | Schematic | Occurrence/births (approx) |
|---|---|---|
| **Ventricular septal defect** A gap between the left and right ventricle allowing blood from the left and right ventricles to mix together | 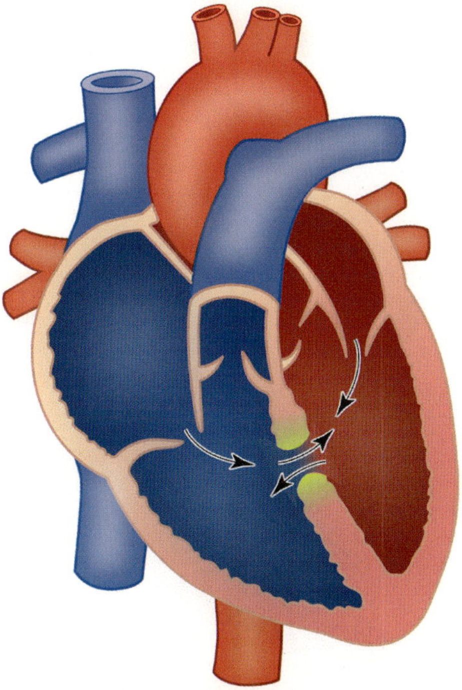 | 1:500 |
| **Pulmonary stenosis** Reduced blood flow to lungs following narrowing of the semilunar valve | 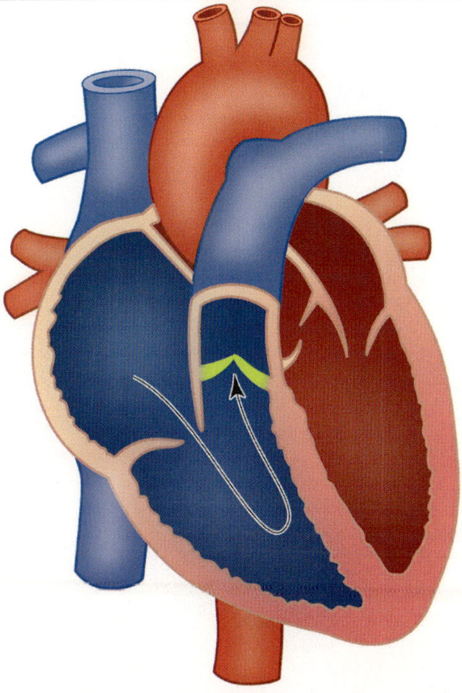 | 1:2,800 |

(continued)

**Table 9.1**  (continued)

| Congenital defect | Schematic | Occurrence/births (approx) |
|---|---|---|
| **Transposition of the great arteries** Essentially pulmonary trunk and the aorta reverse their normal locations resulting in oxygenated blood moving around pulmonary system while de-oxygenated blood moves around the systemic circuit | Aorta Pulmonary trunk | 1:1,000 |
| **Tetralogy of Fallot** Narrowing of pulmonary trunk, pulmonary valve stenosis, ventricular septal defect and aortic opening in both ventricles leading to RVH | | 1:2,000 |

## Patent Foramen Ovale

The function of fossa ovalis has been discussed in Chap. 1. To recap: The fossa ovalis is the remains of what was once a hole (foramen) that existed between the left atrium and the right atrium, located in the atrial septum (Fig. 9.2). This hole allows blood to bypass the lungs in a developing fetus when fetal oxygen supply is provided via the placenta, as the fetal lungs are undeveloped. In some cases the fossa ovalis fails to close and can allow blood to pass from the right to left atrium, this can be due to increased intrathoracic pressure, resulting from coughing, sneezing or trying to pass stool. This condition is referred to as a Patent Foramen Ovale or PFO. A PFO can lead to a stroke or heart attack if a clot passes from the right to left atrium.

## Patent Ductus Arteriosus (PDA)

The ductus arteriosus connects the aorta and pulmonary artery (Fig. 9.3). Pressure forces blood from the aorta to the pulmonary artery as aortic pressure is higher than pulmonary pressure. This in turn increases blood flow through the left side of the

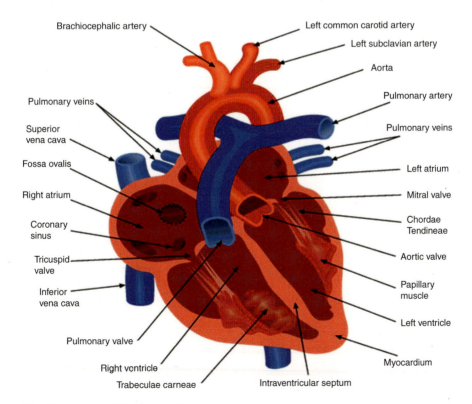

**Fig. 9.2** Location of the Fossa ovalis

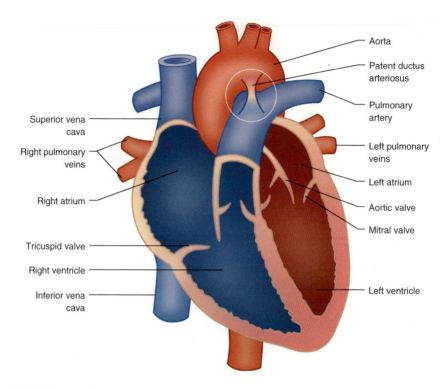

**Fig. 9.3** A patent ductus arteriosus (PDA)

heart. This can cause left atrial abnormality and/or left ventricular hypertrophy. An increase in PR interval can also sometimes be seen on the ECG, although rarely seen with adults. Large PDA's can manifest as biventricular hypertrophy on the ECG. In contrast if the PDA is small the ECG could be completely normal.

## Tetralogy of Fallot

Is a rare congenital condition that encompasses several cardiac defects, including: narrowing of the pulmonary trunk, pulmonary valve stenosis, ventricular septal defect and the aorta being positioned directly over the ventricular septal defect, often termed an overriding aorta. The principal problems associated with tetralogy of Fallot arise due to the pulmonary stenosis and ventricular septal defect (see Fig. 9.4).

Most cases are picked up when a baby is born. Low blood oxygen levels can cause the newborn to appear cyanosed, an echocardiogram usually confirms the condition. Surgery in the form of a major repair operation is often used to correct this condition with a good statistical outcome. As the child grows following

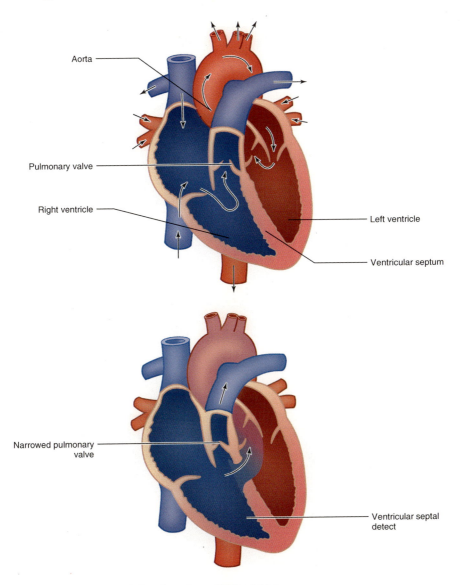

**Fig. 9.4** A normal heart (*left*) and tetralogy of Fallot (*right*)

surgery there will be a degree of pulmonary regurgitation as blood passes back into the right ventricle, due to the abnormal pulmonary valve that doesn't close properly. Over time this can lead to right ventricular hypertrophy. Tetralogy of Fallot can also be associated with Down's syndrome and a syndrome called 22q11 deletion. The ECG findings of tetralogy of Fallot can include right axis deviation, voltage criteria for right ventricular hypertrophy and dominant R waves in the precordial leads.

## Atrial Septal Defect (ASD)

Is a congenital defect in the interatrial septum separating the left and right atrium. This defect allows blood to flow between the two chambers. The mixing of oxygenated and deoxygenated blood can lower the oxygen levels in arterial blood. There are different subcategories of ASD, including, PFO, Ostium primum and ostium secundum atrial septal defects (Fig. 9.5); ostium secundum is the most common type of ASD and may show right axis deviation, whereas an ostium primum shows a left axis deviation. A complete or incomplete right bundle branch block is usually seen with ASD's.

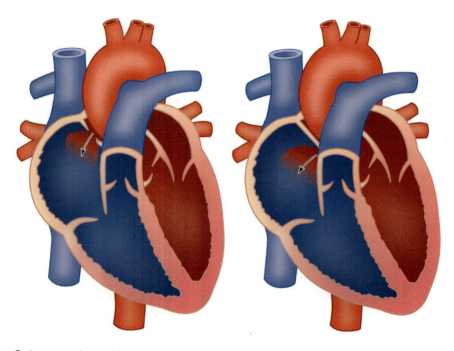

Ostium secundum atrial septal defect

Possible ECG findings:

- RBBB
- Normal or right axis deviation
- 1st Degree AV block
- Right atrial abnormality
- Notching of R waves in inferior leads
- AF or Atrial Flutter (in adults)

Ostium primum atrial septal defect

Possible ECG findings:

- RBBB (complete or incomplete)
- Left axis deviation
- 1st Degree AV block
- Left atrial abnormality

**Fig. 9.5**  An ostium secundum and primum ASD

## Ventricular Septal Defect (VSD)

Work in the same way as ASD's but affect the interventricular septum. There are also various subtypes of VSD. ECG findings can include; Right and left atrial abnormalities, RVH/LVH, RBBB (complete or incomplete) and Katz-Wachtel sign. Katz-Wachtel sign or phenomenon was first described in the late 1930s. It describes tall biphasic RS complexes in leads $V_2$, $V_3$ or $V_4$ of a minimum height of 50 mm.

## Coarctation of Aorta

This is essentially a narrowing of part of the aorta (see Fig. 9.6). This often affects the blood supply to the lower portion of the body. As the heart has to work harder to force blood through the narrowed section of the aorta the patients blood pressure may increase. Sometimes the patient may be hypertensive in the upper body, conversely they can also be hypotensive in the lower body. Due to the increase in

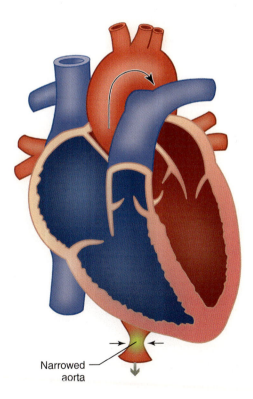

**Fig. 9.6** Coarctation of the aorta

Narrowed aorta

ventricular workload the patient may also develop left ventricular hypertrophy. If the aortic narrowing is severe the condition will usually be picked up in early life and lead to heart failure if untreated. If the narrowing is not severe the condition may not be detected until later in life. Coarctation of the aorta can be treated by surgically removing the narrowed section of aorta and performing an anastomosis, or by less invasive balloon angioplasty.

ECG features of Coarctation of aorta can include: Voltage criteria for left ventricular hypertrophy, left atrial abnormality, first degree AV nodal block and a right bundle branch block (either complete or incomplete).

## Ebstein's Anomaly

A congenital deformity of the tricuspid valve leaflets (Fig. 9.7). This abnormality leads to tricuspid regurgitation, which in turn can lead to right atrial enlargement. Symptoms include: cyanosis, dyspnoea, heart failure, ventricular arrhythmias and SVT. Wolff-Parkinson-White syndrome is often associated with the anomaly (found in around 50 % of cases). Other abnormalities are often found in conjunction with Ebstein's, including; ASD and PFO.

Ebstein's anomaly is relatively rare and accounts for less than 1 % of congenital cardiac disease. Echocardiography provides the definitive diagnosis for Ebstein's anomaly. The ECG may reveal signs of right atrial enlargement, complete or incomplete RBBB, first degree AV block and small R waves in $V_1$ and $V_2$. T-wave inversion is sometimes seen in $V_1$–$V_4$. Tricuspid valve repair or replacement surgery is frequently utilized to good effect.

## Transposition of the Great Arteries

This describes a condition where the aorta and the pulmonary trunk are transposed (change places). Oxygenated blood moves around the pulmonary system, while de-oxygenated blood moves around the systemic circuit. This condition is also associated with other abnormalities, such as; VSD, ASD and PDA. The condition is more common when the mother suffers a viral illness, alcoholism, is diabetic or aged over 40 years while pregnant. It is also worth noting that transposition of the great arteries is a subgroup of transposition of the great vessels, which can involve the transposition of any of the greater vessels, including: inferior vena cava, aorta, and the pulmonary veins/artery. ECG findings can be difficult to discern and may look like an inferior MI due to ventricular inversion and inversion of the bundle branches, leading to right to left septal activation. Q waves can sometimes be seen in the right precordial leads. AV blocks are also commonly seen.

**Fig. 9.7** Normal heart (*left*), Ebstein's anomaly (*right*)

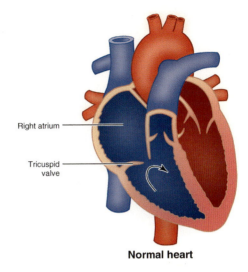

**Normal heart**

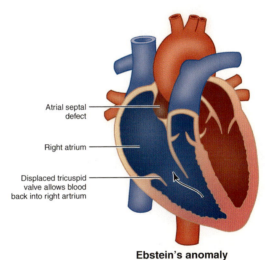

**Ebstein's anomaly**

## Dextrocardia

Can be described as a congenital defect in which the heart is located on the right side of the body instead of the left. ECG features of dextrocardia can include: Inverted P waves in lead I, right axis deviation, QRS complexes get progressively smaller in leads $V_1$–$V_6$. Lead aVR may also be positively deflected (Fig. 9.8). To obtain a meaningful ECG when faced with a patient with dextrocardia the practitioner should swap the right and left arm leads over and place the chest leads on the

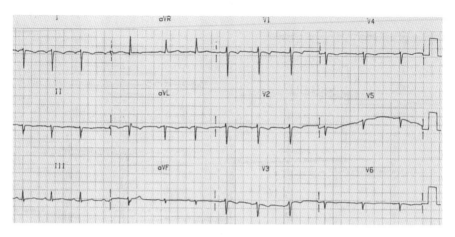

**Fig. 9.8** Dextrocardia [Life in the Fast Lane (http://lifeinthefastlane.com/education/procedures/
lead-positioning/)/CC BY-SA 4.0 (http://creativecommons.org/licenses/by-sa/4.0/)]

opposite side of the chest in a mirror image to how they would normally be applied
(carrying out a right sided ECG is discussed in Chap. 7). There are several subtypes
of dextrocardia:

## Isolated Dextrocardia/Dextrocardia of Embryonic Arrest

The heart is positioned far to the right of the thorax and can be associated with other
serious cardiac abnormalities.

## Dextrocardia Situs Inversus

This is essentially a mirror image of the heart on the left but on the right hand side
of the thorax. Other abdominal organs may also appear in mirror positions to their
normal counterparts.

## Technical Dextrocardia

This is essentially an error in the recording of the ECG in which a patient with their
heart in the normal position can appear to have an ECG recording similar to that
found in a dextrocardia patient. This is caused by the practitioner accidently

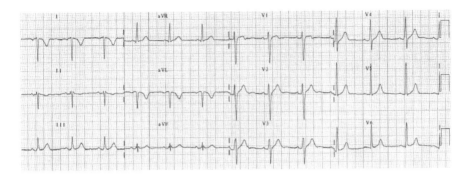

**Fig. 9.9** Technical dextrocardia

swapping the limb leads over. The main way to tell the difference between a real dextrocardia and a technical dextrocardia is the R wave progression, which is usually normal in technical dextrocardia. Another clue can be found by examining any previous ECG's the patient has which would obviously look different if they were previously normal (especially lead aVR). After recording an ECG the practitioner should always check to see to see that the ECG has been recorded correctly (Fig. 9.9).

## Congenital Accessory Pathways

Extra pathways in the heart that some people are born with can allow impulses to travel back up the conduction system leading to a sustained tachycardia. Wolff-Parkinson-White syndrome (WPW) is one such example. WPW and congenital accessory pathways are discussed in more detail in Chap. 6.

## Normal Child ECG Values

There are many differences between the adult ECG and the pediatric ECG, the majority of which are seen in the first year of life. When looking at the ECG of a child or adolescent it is important to be aware of some of the key differences between what are considered normal findings in an adults ECG and what is considered normal in a childs ECG. The heart rate is a key example of this. The younger the child the higher the heart rate. Chart 9.1 shows the upper and lower limits of a childs heart rate based on their age. The mean or average rate is displayed on the chart in yellow. As the child ages the heart rate decreases moving towards the adult average by age 12–16 years.

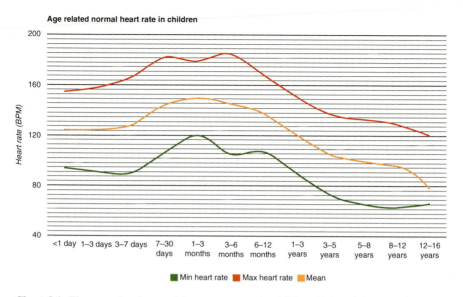

**Chart 9.1** The age related normal heart rates seen in children (Adapted from Davignon A, Rautaharju P, Boisselle E, et al. Normal ECG standards for infants and children. Pediatr Cardiol. 1979/1980;1:133–52)

In an adult a heart rate as high as an infants would indicated a tachycardia and require treatment. In the infant however this is entirely normal and is caused by the lower cardiac output, caused in turn by a lower stroke volume. Conversely a normal adult heart rate seen in an infant can be seen as a pathological bradycardia. The higher heart rate helps to compensate for this reduced output. This can also be said for other features of the pediatric ECG, which compared with that an adult would point to an abnormality. In newborns the right ventricle is larger than the left. This affects the appearance of the ECG and the QRS axis.

There will usually be positively deflected QRS complexes in the precordial leads and aVR showing the right sided dominance (see Fig. 9.10).

## *Axis*

The ECG changes rapidly in the newborn and correct interpretation can be affected by age. In the newborn the right ventricle is dominant owing to the high pulmonary arterial pressure in utero. This has an impact on the cardiac axis with newborns showing right axis deviation. In the first few years of life, the left ventricle increases in size becoming dominant, causing an axis shift to the normal adult axis (Chart 9.2).

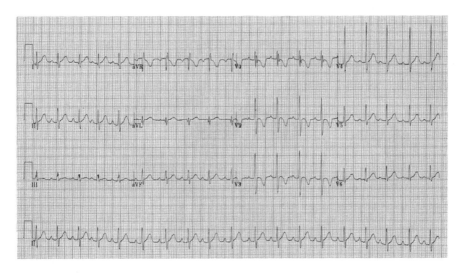

**Fig. 9.10** A normal pediatric ECG taken from a 2 year old male [Life in the Fast Lane (http://lifein-thefastlane.com/education/procedures/lead-positioning/)/CC BY-SA 4.0 (http://creativecommons.org/licenses/by-sa/4.0/)]

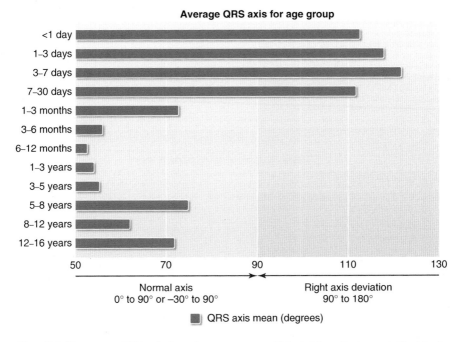

**Chart 9.2** The average QRS axis dependent on age group (Adapted from Davignon A, Rautaharju P, Boisselle E, et al. Normal ECG standards for infants and children. Pediatr Cardiol. 1979/1980;1:133–52)

## *Intervals/ST Segment*

The PR interval also differs depending on the age (Chart 9.3) and is normally shorter in children than adults. As a result of the shorter PR interval AV conduction delays may be present (Table 9.2). The duration of the QRS complex is also shorter in children than adults (Table 9.3). It is speculated that this could pertain to the smaller cardiac muscle mass found in the young. As with the adult, the QT interval is dependent on the heart rate and is corrected for (QTc formula). The QTc is often higher in children than adults, with the upper normal limit being around 440 ms. T waves are variable, often upright for the first week of life before becoming negative in $V_1$ and positive in $V_5$–$V_6$. Any ST elevation of 1 mm or more above the baseline is abnormal in newborns.

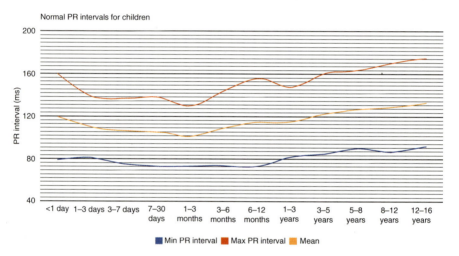

**Chart 9.3** Normal age related child PR intervals (Adapted from Davignon A, Rautaharju P, Boisselle E, et al. Normal ECG standards for infants and children. Pediatr Cardiol. 1979/1980;1:133–52)

| **Table 9.2** Normal rhythm variations in children | AV nodal heart blocks (first Degree AV block, second Degree AV block Type I) |
|---|---|
| | Sinus arrhythmia |
| | Short sinus pauses |
| | Premature atrial or ventricular beats |

**Table 9.3** Age related QRS duration

| Age group | QRS duration ($V_5$) in seconds |
|---|---|
| 0–1 days | 0.02–0.08 |
| 1–3 days | 0.02–0.07 |
| 3–7 days | 0.02–0.07 |
| 7–30 days | 0.02–0.08 |
| 1–3 months | 0.02–0.08 |

Adapted from Davignon A, Rautaharju P, Boisselle E, et al. Normal ECG standards for infants and children. Pediatr Cardiol. 1979/1980;1:133–52

## Summary of Key Points

- Interpretation of the pediatric ECG is largely dependent on the childs age.
- The right side of the heart is dominant in newborns.
- The heart rate of children and newborns is higher than that of an adult and this is normal.
- There are many congenital conditions that can affect the structure and function of the heart. Most of which are usually discovered in the patients early years of life, however milder defects can first present with symptoms affecting quality of life in adulthood.
- Practitioners should always check ECGs when recording them to ensure correct lead placement to avoid technical dextrocardia.
- Patients with dextrocardia require that the ECG is recorded with leads in mirror image to their usual position to gain a meaningful recording.

## Quiz

Q1. Which side of the heart shows dominance in the newborn?

    (A) Left
    (B) Right

Q2. A Patent Foramen Ovale or PFO is…

    (A) A normal developmental stage in cardiac development
    (B) The fossa ovalis failing to close as the heart develops allowing blood to pass from the right to left atrium
    (C) A gap between the two ventricles

Q3. The main difference between technical and true dextrocardia is…

    (A)  In technical dextrocardia the R wave progression is usually normal.
    (B)  In technical dextrocardia large R waves are seen in leads $V_2$ and $V_4$
    (C)  In technical dextrocardia P waves are always positively defected in lead I

Q4. A heart rate of 110 bpm in a 6 month old child is…

    (A)  A sign of tachycardia requiring additional tests and investigations
    (B)  A bradycardia requiring urgent treatment
    (C)  A normal finding in a child of that age

Q5. Which subtype of dextrocardia describes the heart being in a mirror position on the right to its usually position on the left?

    (A)  Dextrocardia situs inversus
    (B)  Technical dextrocardia
    (C)  Isolated dextrocardia/dextrocardia of embryonic arrest

Q6. A newborn child is likely to show signs of right axis deviation on the ECG

    (A)  True
    (B)  False

Answers: Q1 = B, Q2 = B, Q3 = A, Q4 = C, Q5 = A, Q6 = A

# Index

© Springer-Verlag London 2015
A. Davies, A. Scott, *Starting to Read ECGs: A Comprehensive Guide to Theory
and Practice*, DOI 10.1007/978-1-4471-4965-1

Printed by Printforce, the Netherlands